D1441991

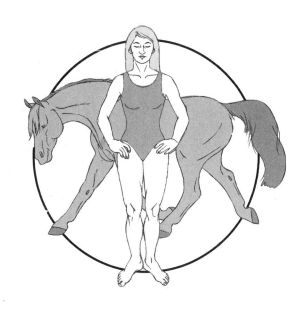

# PILATES FOR THE
# DRESSAGE RIDER

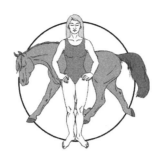

# PILATES FOR THE DRESSAGE RIDER

ENGAGING THE HUMAN SPINE USING PILATES

BY

JANICE DULAK

Musculoskeletal system by Katrin Haselbacher, PT
Photographs by Andrew Ducette
Illustrations by Eva Sandor

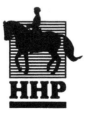

Half Halt Press, Inc.
Boonsboro, Maryland

# PILATES FOR THE DRESSAGE RIDER
## ENGAGING THE HUMAN SPINE USING PILATES
© 2006 JANICE DULAK

Published in the United States of America by
Half Halt Press, Inc.
P.O.Box 67
Boonsboro, MD 21713

All rights reserved. No Part of this book may be reproduced in any way or by any means without permission in writing from the publisher.

Book and Jacket Design by Jim Farber
Illustrations by Eva Sandor
Photographs by Andy Ducette

Library of Congress Cataloging-in-Publication Data

Dulak, Janice.
   Pilates for the dressage rider : engaging the human spine using pilates / by Janice Dulak ; musculoskeletal system by Katrin Haselbacher ; photographs by Andrew Ducette ; illustrations by Eva Sandor.
      p. cm.
   Includes bibliographical references.
   ISBN 0-939481-72-3
   1. Pilates method. 2. Dressage. I. Title.
   RA781.4.D85 2006
   613.7'1--dc22

                        2006021352

# DEDICATION

*This book is dedicated to my mother, whose creative mind was always seeking ways to make things work, and to my father, for instilling in me a great love of horses.*

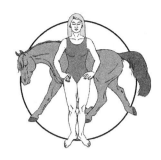

# TABLE OF CONTENTS

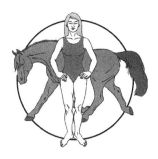

# ACKNOWLEDGMENTS AND THANKS

My special thanks go to Romana, who carries the Pilates torch and has taught me all I know about Pilates. I am forever honored to have my husband John at my side, who always supports me, even when I leap without really looking. I also want to acknowledge India, (aka: Super Hoofer,) my first horse who refused to trail ride or jump, forcing me to find dressage.

A special thanks to the following people who have specifically helped me in this endeavor:

Katrin Haselbacher, Noël Chase, Barbara Geissler, Leslie Driesner

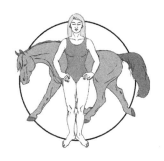

# ILLUSTRATIONS

## CHAPTER 6

FIGURE 6

1. CORRECT MOUNTED POSITION

2. SPINE STRETCH FORWARD

3. LEG LIFTS—CORRECT

4. LEG LIFTS—INCORRECT

5. SIDE BEND

6. TWISTING

7. ARCHING—CORRECT

8. ARCHING—INCORRECT

## CHAPTER 7

FIGURE 7

1. CONCEPTUAL VERSION OF THE OPEN LEG ROCKER POSITION WHILE MOUNTED

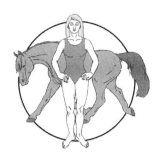

# INTRODUCTION

In December 1993, I was given my first horse, a thoroughbred straight off the track. Having been horse crazy as a kid watching the Kentucky Derby every year with my father, being given a thoroughbred was as close to heaven as I could imagine. I was a professional modern dancer, teaching dance at Stephens College in Columbia, Missouri and had just been certified in Pilates. Used to being in complete control of my body, when I began to ride this horse, I quickly realized that I had no clue about what I was doing. I took hunt seat and then dressage lessons, which gave me my first insight into real riding. However as the years passed, I realized the more I learned about riding, the less I actually knew. This, of course, is true of most disciplines; however, after a while, it began to make no sense to me whatsoever. With all the movement skill I possessed from my years of dance and Pilates training, I still did not understand how to use an independent seat, legs and hands, nor could I figure out how to execute a half halt. Frustrated, I wondered if I ever could become as graceful and effective on my horse as I had been when performing a duet on stage.

I began to read voraciously trying to figure things out. I subscribed to magazines, checked books out of the library and slowly became even more confused. I took more lessons and clinics. Everyone had a different way of describing a half halt, how to effectively turn, stop, perform an upward transition, etc. Although I was humbled by the difficulty of learning the discipline of dressage, with my past dance accomplishments, I felt that I just couldn't be that difficult to teach. Somehow I felt there had to be a more efficient way to learn to ride with the elegance and grace of the upper-level riders.

Meanwhile, the Pilates work that had invigorated my professional dance career began to inform my teaching as I started understanding how Pilates principles and concepts could relate to dancing. As with riding, dance for beginners is also confusing. Mysterious phrases such as "lift up," "use your arms from your back" and "use your center" are thrown at dancers, but there are rarely any explanations of what the phrases mean or how to perform them. I finally began to see how specific Pilates exercises could be used to explain these mysterious phrases to my dancers and my teaching style changed dramatically. The once-befuddled dancers were now making quicker progress, as they understood how to turn a phrase such as "lift up" into a clear and precise movement of the body.

Besides Pilates, dressage also crept in to my dance teaching as I slowly began to understand how getting a horse on the bit was really all about the engagement of the underside of the horse, stretching over the topline. This concept is also true for dancers: unless they engage their abdominals correctly to keep their spines lengthened, dancers will lift their chins and hollow their backs. With this posture, the movement is not truly coming from their centers, but rather from their arms and legs. It was not unusual for me to teach my dancers by getting down on all fours to demonstrate how, if they didn't use their Pilates skills when they worked, they would look like a sway-backed horse. In this posture, the movement would not have a dancing aesthetic or the power and energy to project to the audience sitting in the balcony of a theater. With both the Pilates and dressage examples, explaining dance technique became quite simple. I also began to see how Pilates exercises, principles and concepts could help me understand how the horse uses his back. Still, riding dressage seemed an insurmountable mystery to me.

Over the years, I slowly began to realize that Pilates, riding, training a horse and dance have an important element in common: each requires that the core of the body be stabilized in order to generate and control the energy from the center into free-flowing movement of the rest of the body. Using the working Pilates principles, the mystery of the "half halt with your body," "use your back," "rounder" and "independent seat and hands" slowly began to make sense. I needed to control the center of my body with my "Pilates Powerhouse" in order to use the correct amount of muscle tension in other parts of my body for my aids to be effective. This was simple! I discovered that the exercises I performed during a Pilates workout, besides being a great conditioning program, also could be used while mounted to achieve that grace and ease of upper-level riders. As a side benefit, through the Pilates exercises, I began to feel how I was using my own spine, which gave me new insight into the riding concepts of being engaged, "on the bit" and lengthening and collection.

The purpose of this book is for the reader/rider to utilize my explorations into how Pilates can help the dressage rider so that it may enhance the rider's ability to succeed in dressage. In order to fulfill this purpose, there are three basic goals: to give the rider an introduction to Pilates and a basic workout to do at home or on the horse, to help the rider understand and gain control over engagement in her own spine, and to guide the rider toward using the knowledge of the body gained by the practice of Pilates to help her find new ways to use her body to improve her riding.

The first goal of this book is designed to give the reader a basic understanding of Pilates principles that will lead to a basic workout, which, in turn, will develop core strength and contribute to proper posture and symmetry of the body. The exercises you will find in Chapter 4 and 5 are pure Pilates. Nothing has been altered or changed in any way. The genius of the body of Joseph Pilates' work remains as he taught and has been carried on by the heir to the method, Romana Kryzanowska. The exercises in this book have been culled from more than 500 Pilates exercises and are chosen to best suit the needs of the dressage rider. These selected exercises are a good introduction to Pilates but, like the dressage horse and rider who move on to more advanced movements, the Pilates practitioner will want to advance in the Pilates Method. Just as the leg yield at First Level begins the concept of lateral work that later evolves into the half pass at Third Level, the Roll Up you perform today will become the Roll Over at the advanced level in Pilates. But like dressage, every advanced movement in Pilates is built on the basics. Mastering the basics is key to furthering work in Pilates. The challenge is to keep true to the quality of the work as the exercises become more complex.

The second goal of this book is for the reader to use the Pilates exercises to understand and feel engagement in her own spine so she can develop an understanding and feel of the same in the horse's spine. Keeping engagement while lengthening and collecting a horse's gaits are concepts often only in the mind of the rider at first. The feel for it often takes years to develop. The work of Joseph Pilates can be described to the rider as the lengthening and collection of the human spine through engagement of the "Powerhouse" muscles. Mastering the basic Pilates exercises in this book will help the rider feel and learn to control the lengthening and collection of her own spine by engagement of her Pilates Powerhouse. It is then my hope that she can more quickly develop the feel for it in her horse.

The third goal is to relate specific muscular actions as performed in a Pilates exercise to the specific body mechanics required to execute dressage movements, thereby de-mystifying the "how to." Just as the "ah-ha's" came to my dancers and myself when a specific Pilates exercise could be used to feel a *cambré* in ballet class, it is my hope that a specific Pilates exercise can help the aspiring dressage rider to feel her body positioning for a shoulder-in and other dressage movements.

Not claiming to be a riding instructor by any means, the suggestions in Chapter 7 are meant as a springboard for the rider's further exploration. As a long-time teacher of dance and Pilates, I have learned that information can be given out and shared, but it is the student who will figure out how the information can be used in her own way. If the suggestions here can lead to a quicker "ah-ha" for just one rider, then the book will have served its purpose.

Just as with dressage training, Pilates is something that improves over time. The Hundreds you perform today will not be the Hundreds you perform a year from now if you continue your workouts: your form will be better, you will have more strength to keep your head up (on the bit), your abdominals will engage more deeply (collection), your spine will be more supple (stretching over the topline) and your buttocks (haunches) will be stronger and legs more flexible (to reach up under yourself).

This book will give you your start in understanding the work of Joseph Pilates. However, just as with all the excellent books on dressage instruction, it will aid your understanding of the work but it can never replace a good instructor. It is my hope that the rider will seek to further her Pilates workout in a studio, one on one, with qualified instruction. In this environment, the student can advance the Pilates conditioning step by step from these basic principles and exercises, moving through the system to the advanced movements.

Simple things are not always easy. Although I will try to present these simple Pilates concepts, I will not say it is easy. It will take time and concentration. I hope this book will help you on your way to become the rider you hope to be.

Happy Hundreds,
*Janice Dulak*

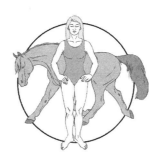

# CHAPTER 1
# WHAT? WHO? WHY?

## WHAT IS PILATES?

Pilates is a body conditioning method that is safe and effective for all ages and body types. Simply put, Pilates is strength and stretch with control. (Couldn't that be a definition of dressage—that the horse be strong and supple and have the ability to control his own body in self-carriage?) With the help of a qualified, certified instructor, a Pilates workout can be gentle enough for a person recovering from hip replacement surgery or an hour of vigorous exercise that can be taxing even for a professional athlete or dancer.

Pilates places equal emphasis on the flexibility and strength in all the muscles of the body and seeks to balance this strength and flexibility in order to create and maintain optimum posture for more efficient body use. Most of the exercises are low impact and non-weight-bearing. Exercise sessions focus on quality of performance rather than quantity or repetition. Fewer and more precise repetitions train the body more efficiently.

Beginning with what is often referred to as "core strength," Pilates requires the practitioner to find the deepest abdominal muscles, which will be detailed in Chapter 2. These muscles combined with the active use of the gluteals, create what Pilates called the "Powerhouse" of movement. Every exercise performed in Pilates demands that the Powerhouse—or center—be engaged to control the movement of all the joints of the body

At first, the range of motion in the joints is kept small so the practitioner can develop and learn to use the Powerhouse to control their use. Through this slow and careful work, the practitioner dynamically develops flexibility. As control over the Powerhouse develops and flexibility in the muscles increases, the range of motion in each joint can be gradually expanded. Exercises become progressively demanding and, at the advanced levels, they ask that the Powerhouse be engaged while flexing, bending, rotating and extending the spine as well as when producing the fullest range of motion possible in all joints of the body.

# WHO WAS JOSEPH PILATES?

Joseph Pilates developed the Pilates Method of Physical and Mental Conditioning (Contrology) over a span of 50 years in the early 1900s. In his words, "Contrology is a complete coordination of the body, mind, and spirit (that) develops the body uniformly, corrects wrong postures, restores physical vitality, and invigorates the mind and elevates the spirit."[1]

Born in Germany, Joseph Pilates immigrated to the United States after a career as a circus tumbler, an acrobatic performer and a fitness instructor for the military police. He opened a gymnasium in New York City in the early 1920's, and it was there that he was able to complete the design for, and patent, the gym equipment that is unique to his method. Pilates explains: "Here the accent is stretching, bending, and tensing the body muscles, and flexing them. You'll notice we have no ropes, no Indian clubs, or any motor-driven gadgets. There are no weights to lift either. Ever see an animal lift weights for fun or exercise?"[2]

Indeed, Pilates often referred to the grace, poise and suppleness of animals when he spoke about his method. He spent a great deal of time during his childhood observing animals, both in the wild and at zoos. Combining his observations with the knowledge he gained from anatomy books he was given as a young boy, he formulated basic concepts for his work, which are to develop strength and flexibility equally in the whole body and gain grace and ease in movement. Romana Kryzanowska, heir to the Pilates Method, states: "The basic goal has remained the same—to lengthen and strengthen all the muscles of the

Figure 1-1 Joseph Pilates assisting a client on the ladder barrel (circa 1960)

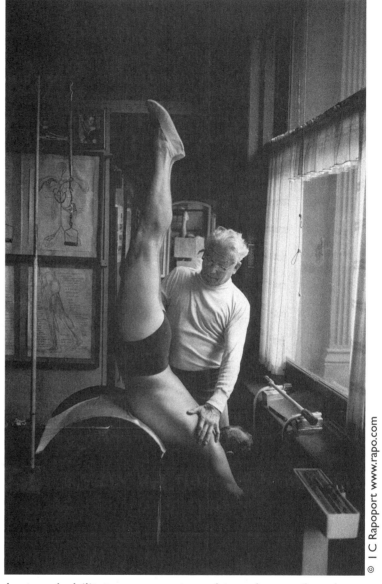

© I C Rapoport www.rapo.com

body into a balanced whole, to rehabilitate or correct, and to enhance the physical efforts of the student."[3]

Joseph and his wife, Clara Pilates, ran his New York studio until he died in the late 1960's. His work was left to Kryzanowska who continues the Pilates tradition with her daughter Sari Mejia Santo and Sari's daughter through Romana's Pilates Inc.

# WHY PILATES?

There are many ways to condition the human body to prepare it for athletic endeavors. However, each sport has unique requirements for body conditioning. The workout for a professional football player is not the workout that would satisfy the needs of the dancer. The work of the marathon runner would not necessarily suit the needs of a sprinter. The dressage rider also has specific conditioning needs that the work of Joseph Pilates meets without reservation.

Riders wanting to become more fit in order to ride better may find that just exercising does not necessarily enhance their ability to ride horses more efficiently. Of course there is a benefit the rider can gain from any type of working out. However, for exercise to improve riding skills, the exercises must be designed to teach the rider how to integrate and utilize the skills gained from working out with the specific use of the musculature required for the art of dressage. For example, a dancer who wants to increase strength for her dancing might gain strength lifting weights. However the strength gained in this manner may not allow for the flexibility needed to integrate the strength in a way that would be conducive to performing specific dance steps. The hours the dancer spends exercising in this way, although beneficial to her well being, does little to help her feel what her body needs to do to execute a pirouette.

In the same sense, a dressage rider who seeks to become more physically fit so that she can ride her horse better may spend hours in the gym. And while she eventually gets stronger and perhaps more flexible, working out in the gym may not really improve her riding skills. Furthermore, the exercise may do little to educate her sense of "feel" for what the horse is doing. For example, if the rider cannot feel engagement in her horse, hours will be spent riding around in circles executing exercises to get the horse round and on the bit. While this will give the horse and rider a workout, it will take longer for the rider to teach the horse to be engaged than if the rider understood the feeling of engagement.

Pilates offers the rider more than just body conditioning to take back to the barn. With the practice of the Pilates Method, she will also find and learn to use her core muscles, which she can apply to her riding skills. She will begin to understand how she might use a specific Pilates exercise to hold her body dynamically while performing a specific dressage movement. With the practice of Pilates, she will also deepen her feel of engagement in herself, which can lead to an understanding and feeling of engagement in her horse.

# THE SIX PRINCIPLES OF PILATES

There are six principles of Pilates that are inherent in practicing the work of Joseph Pilates. Although all principles are required in all exercises, in the beginning, I guide practitioners toward the first three: centering, concentration and control. As the practitioner moves "up the training scale," precision, flow and breath become important and are emphasized as control over the exercises allow.

## CENTERING

Work in Pilates requires that all movement initiate from the Powerhouse of the body outward to the extremities. The Powerhouse, as Pilates called it, can be described simply as the band around the midsection of the body. More specifically, it is the deep abdominal and gluteal muscles, which work in conjunction with the upper thighs and low back muscles (See Chapter 2). Their strengthening and use are the priority of all Pilates exercises. Also inherent in this first principle is attention to the centerline of the body. Drawing a line down the center of the body, the trunk (or as Pilates called it, the "Box") should be symmetrical (See Chapter 2). Each exercise requires the practitioner to not only work from the Powerhouse, but also be cognizant of working symmetrically so the muscles are working and developing evenly. This leads to correction of muscle imbalances that can cause skeletal deviations leading to poor posture and inefficient use of the body.

## CONCENTRATION

Joseph Pilates stated: "It is the mind that guides the body." All Pilates exercises require the full participation of the body and mind. The practitioner will use the strength and control of one set of muscles to lengthen and stretch the opposing set of muscles. While doing this, she must be aware of the Powerhouse and the symmetry of the Box at all times. This dynamic work requires extreme mental focus. This practice of concentration can help one become aware of how the whole body is (or is not) involved while performing any task. For example, one often loses awareness of the control over Powerhouse while executing a side bend. Doing this repeatedly can result in habitual improper form, which, eventually, can cause strain on structures in the lower back—joints, ligaments, discs, as well as muscles. Pilates requires full concentration to discipline the mind and body so the work is true and correct.

## CONTROL

From the practice of centering and concentration comes control over the body, which is why Pilates called his method of exercising "Contrology." Pilates develops the understanding and practice of control by integrating the mind and the body while exercising. What may appear to be an exercise for the leg requires control of the Powerhouse and symmetry of the Box as well as the studied use of the arms and head. Using the Powerhouse to control movement allows for safe and efficient use of the body, which helps in injury prevention.

Precision, flow and breath are the next principles that a practitioner of Pilates will come to understand and use in a Pilates workout. These principles fine-tune the exercises so the advanced work looks seemingly effortless and graceful.

## PRECISION

Joseph Pilates believed the body could be fine-tuned by exercising with accurate form and fewer repetitions. Work in this way leads to the maximum effect with the minimum of effort. With the practice of Pilates, the body becomes more toned and aware, able to respond to minute directions or corrections. Devoting concentration to precision becomes life-long work and the discipline of Pilates.

## FLOW

Free-flowing movement of the body with strength and dynamics within the exercise and during transitions from exercise to exercise is the goal of every Pilates workout. To watch an advanced Pilates workout is a study in grace, ease, poise and beauty of movement. Here the practitioner has learned to allow the energy to emanate from the center of the body and flow to the extremities without blockage by excess mental or muscular tension. Pilates helps the practitioner understand relaxation within movements that require strength and also gives the practitioner the strength to afford this ease of movement.

## BREATH

All Pilates exercises done correctly require rhythm and breath. Each exercise has a deep breathing pattern with the emphasis on the exhalation. The use of breath helps create the dynamics and rhythm for each exercise. Breathing deeply encourages relaxation in the muscles allowing the body to elongate and move with grace and ease. Learning to use the breath during moments of physical exertions can help the body remain strong but relaxed. The rhythm and dynamics of an exercise in Pilates often can be defined by the practitioner's breathing pattern to help the movement flow. In Pilates, the inhalation is often on the effort and the exhalation on the stretch or relaxation. By learning to breathe in this way, the practitioner can breathe more fully during moments of physical taxation when she usually tends to hold her breath.

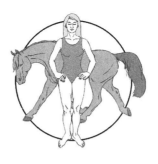

## CHAPTER 2

# PILATES
# AND THE MUSCULOSKELETAL SYSTEM

In the following chapters you will learn Pilates exercises that will improve your core strength, flexibility and posture, and ultimately also help with your performance on a horse. The goal of this chapter is threefold: First, to explain what core and trunk or "powerhouse" and "box" actually mean. Second, to explain why the three hallmarks of Pilates—core strength, good posture and muscle flexibility—are so important. Third, to give you a better sense of key muscles used in Pilates.

## THE POWERHOUSE AND BOX EXPLAINED

### THE CORE

The term "Core" describes the center, middle or midpoint of an object. Like the core of an apple, the core of the human body is its center. Pilates focuses on the core and refers to it simply as the Powerhouse. Definitions of the anatomical borders as well as the muscles of the human core vary. In this book, we define the core as the area from the inner thighs and pelvis up to the lower border of the ribcage. Among the muscles specifically targeted by the method are the following powerhouse muscles: the lower layers of the abdominals, the buttocks, the inner thigh muscles and the small lower-back muscles.

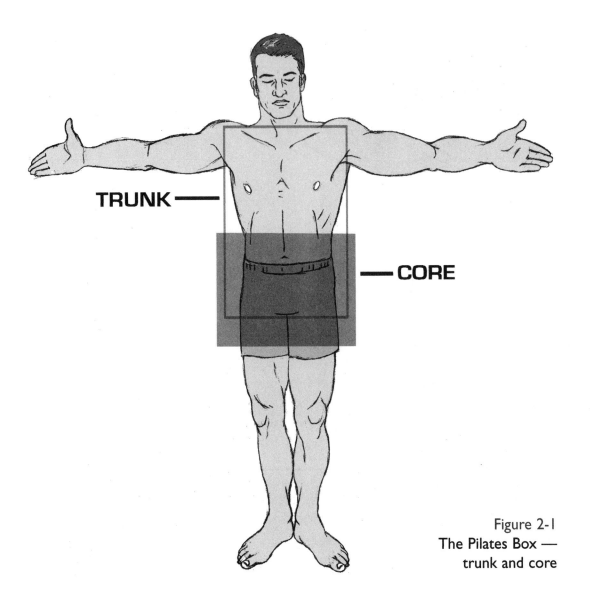

TRUNK

CORE

Figure 2-1
The Pilates Box —
trunk and core

## THE TRUNK

The trunk, or torso, is anatomically defined as the body without the limbs, neck and head. Important muscles of the trunk include the long back muscles, the mid and upper layers of abdominals and the mid and lower trapezius. The trunk also includes the core muscles. In Pilates, the trunk is referred to as the Pilates Box and is essential when referring to posture.

# CORE STRENGTH, GOOD POSTURE AND MUSCLE FLEXIBILITY

Core strength, good posture and muscle flexibility significantly contribute to a healthy musculoskeletal system—meaning that they help the body's structures function efficiently. Non-optimal function requires more energy for movement and can lead to musculoskeletal discomfort, pain and possible injuries. A strong core, flexible muscles (i.e. muscles that have an optimal length to function properly) and good posture contribute to improved performance in physical endeavors.

## CORE STRENGTH

The core provides a stable base for the limbs to generate force and motion. The relationship between the muscles of the core and the limbs has been studied in detail. The results showed that the transversus abdominis was activated involuntarily even before the person lifted the arm.[4] This demonstrates how important the role of the core is for the use of arms and legs. Therefore actively strengthening the core muscles through exercise helps the body function more efficiently.

The core is also important in sports medicine and rehabilitation of injuries. For example, a pitcher uses the core to deliver a powerful pitch. If the pitcher incurs a shoulder injury, core strengthening will be used as an important part of the rehabilitation process. This will allow the athlete to return to the sport more quickly and successfully. Therefore, core strengthening should be incorporated into the rehabilitation of injured arms and legs.

## POSTURE

Good posture means that the body is erect with correct alignment of the bones and joints. Consider a person with optimum posture as in Figure 2-2. Bones and joints are considered well-aligned if the head, the thorax, the pelvis and the legs lie close to an imaginary plumb line drawn from the ears to the ankle. This line should run straight down from the ear through the midpoint of the shoulder, the hip and the knee to the ankle without any deviations. Core and trunk muscles work together to maintain an erect posture against gravity. If the involved

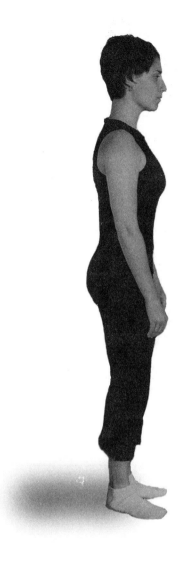

Figure 2-2
Optimum Posture

core and trunk muscles weaken, shorten or are too long and overstretched, they will create deviations from the plumb line, resulting in poor posture. Deviations from the imaginary plumb line, as depicted in Figure 2-3, lead to stress or strain in joints, tendons and ligaments. This stress or strain over an extended period of time will enhance the likelihood of joint wear, possible injury and pain.

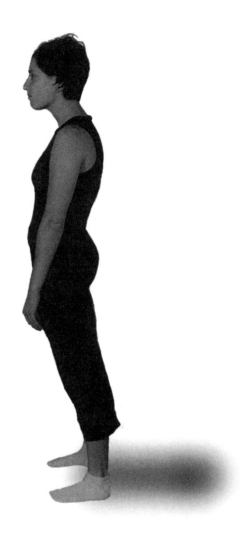

Figure 2-3
Poor Posture

## MUSCLE FLEXIBILITY

Flexibility in muscles implies that a muscle can move through its normal range
of motion. Proper muscle length (not too long and not too short) in a single
muscle is important for optimal function. However, there must also be a balance between the muscle groups that function around a joint for its efficient
use. A muscle imbalance occurs when certain muscles are too weak or too
strong and/or too short or too long in relation to others. For example, the muscles that bend an arm and the muscles that straighten an arm require both opti-

mal length and strength individually, but also in relation to each other. Too little as well as too much flexibility in muscles can cause problems.

A lack of muscle flexibility, which means that muscles are shortened and typically weakened, affects posture and function of joints. Shortened muscles could place the joint in a position that deviates from the norm. A joint can become stiff if the flexibility of the surrounding muscles has decreased. A combination of shortened muscles, bad posture and inefficient body movements can eventually lead to injury. For example, a shortened hip-flexor muscle combined with weakened gluteal muscles lead to a so-called anterior pelvic tilt. This means the front (anterior) top of the pelvis is tilted forward and the tailbone is tipped backwards, increasing the arch of the lower back, as indicated in Figure 2-3. This posture puts the abdominal muscles in a stretched position, making it difficult for them to work properly. This imbalance of overstretched abdominals, weakened gluteal muscles and shortened hip-flexor muscles leads to increased stress and strain in the lower back and results in increased risk of injury.

On the other hand, there can be too much flexibility. This occurs if a joint can be moved beyond normal limits without undue force and discomfort. Such joints are called hypermobile. Hypermobility can affect just one joint (e.g. the knees) or multiple joints. Consider the example of standing with hyperextended knees as shown in Figure 2-3 and sitting as shown in Figure 3-5. In this position the knees are stabilized mainly by the ligaments and no longer by the muscles. This form of joint stabilization puts undue stress on the ligaments and the knee joint. As a result, the anterior thigh muscle (quadriceps), which would normally stabilize the knee joint, weakens because it is not used for the stabilizing function. Furthermore this stance further affects the pelvis, resulting in poor posture.

# INTERPLAY OF CORE STRENGTH, POSTURE AND MUSCLE FLEXIBILITY

The above considerations make it clear that the different aspects of a healthy musculoskeletal system are intertwined. As outlined above, poor posture, abnormal muscle length and weak core/trunk muscles will affect the way a person moves her or his body and the efficiency of those movements. A person with optimal posture, core strength and flexible muscles will perform movements more efficiently and with less energy than a person with deficiencies in those areas.

What are the specific considerations for equestrians? A strong core/trunk is required for the equestrian to maintain an erect posture on the horse. The core/trunk provides stability on a mobile surface (horseback) and counteracts the dynamic forces of the horse's gait that act on the equestrian's body. Equestrians usually have fairly good postures because their postural muscles have adapted to the forces that they encounter during riding. However this does not necessarily mean that their core muscles are strong and that their muscles are flexible. Lack of flexibility can lead to non-optimal body mechanics and can result in musculoskeletal discomfort and eventually, injury. Also, the horse might sense the lack of flexibility or stiffness as increased tension. Therefore it is essential for equestrians to have a strong core, good posture and muscle flexibility in order to maintain a strong but supple position on the horse.

# KEY MUSCLES USED IN PILATES EXERCISES

The following paragraphs should give you a better understanding of the key muscles that are pertinent to the Pilates Powerhouse and Box. These key muscles include the transversus abdominis, the multifidi, the gluteus maximus and buttock muscles, the hip adductors and the mid and lower trapezius muscles.

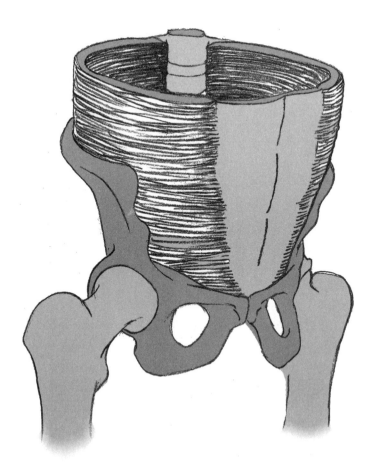

Figure 2-4
Transversus abdominis

## TRANSVERSUS ABDOMINIS

The tranversus abdominis muscle is the deepest abdominal muscle. It expands horizontally around the trunk. The muscle attachments include the lower ribs, a thick tendon plate in the mid and lower back, and the pelvis. The transversus abdominis acts as a corset by flattening the abdominal wall and increasing pressure within the abdomen when contracted. Through the tendon plate the muscle is indirectly attached to the spine and, when activated, provides stability of the trunk and core. A strong transversus abdominis is important for a strong core and as support for the lower back. Weakness of the muscle can cause bulging of the abdomen (as described above in section on posture), which is likely to lead to an increase in low-back arching, as illustrated in Figure 2-3.

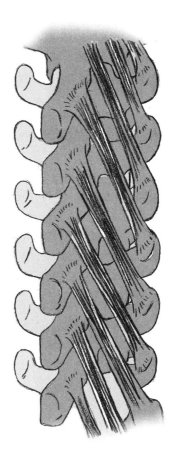

Figure 2-5
Section of Multifidi

## MULTIFIDI

The multifidi are small muscles that extend over two or three vertebrae each along the entire spine. In a healthy individual, the multifidi work in co-activation with the transversus abdominis. The multifidi constitute the deepest layer of spine muscles and provide stability to the spinal vertebrae and ultimately to the whole spine with muscle activation. Conversely, the large torque-producing muscles are generally further away from joints. For example, the long superficial postural back muscles extend all along the back from pelvis to neck. They are important for an erect posture against gravity, but do not provide the same stability to the spine as the multifidi.

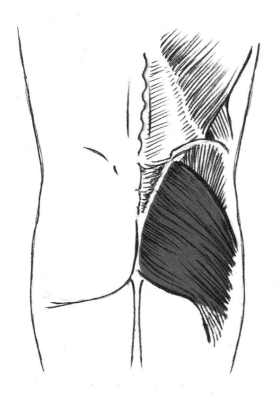

Figure 2-6
Gluteus maximus

## GLUTEUS MAXIMUS/BUTTOCK MUSCLES/HIP ADDUCTORS

The simultaneous activation of the gluteus maximus, external rotators of the hip and inner thigh muscles is required for most Pilates exercises. For example, the stance used in Pilates, which is heels together and toes slightly apart, requires the simultaneous activation of these muscles. See Figure 2-7.

The gluteus maximus is the big muscle that defines the buttock cheek. It is a very important muscle for core stability and good posture. The gluteus maximus has two functions at the hip: extension and external rotation. Other buttock muscles lie below the gluteus maximus and are also used in performing Pilates exercises. Location and orientation of the muscle fibers of these buttock muscles determine their function. It is beyond the scope of this chapter to describe these other buttock muscles. We simplify the buttock muscles into extensors and external rotators of the hip.

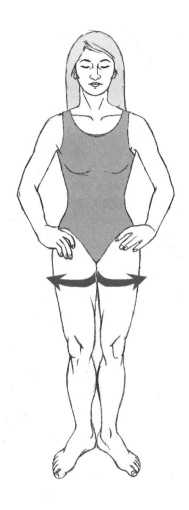

Figure 2-7
**Stance used in Pilates, "engaging the bottom," and "wrapping the thighs"**

Hip extension is the action at the hip when the thigh moves behind the body. It can be exemplified by someone lying flat on the stomach and lifting one leg straight toward the ceiling. Weak hip extensors can create a forward (or anterior) tilt of the pelvis, which can contribute to poor posture.

External rotators of the hip are activated if, for example, a person turns both feet outwards from the hip. Charlie Chaplin made this position famous with his feet-outwards stance and walk. To get into this "Charlie Chaplin position," one has to fully engage the external rotators.

Hip adductors are the muscles on the inside of the thighs. Their main function is to bring the inner thighs together.

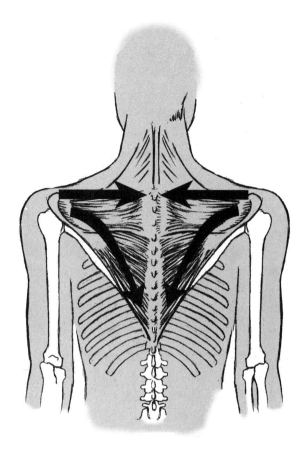

Figure 2-8
Trapezius—mid and lower

## TRAPEZIUS MUSCLE

The trapezius muscle covers the back of the neck and the area between the shoulder blades. Anatomically, it is divided into three different sections because of the different orientations of the muscle fibers. The three sections originate in the back of the head and neck, the upper and thoracic vertebrae, and the mid- to lower-thoracic vertebrae, respectively. The three sections converge to insert on the shoulder blade at different locations.

The origins and insertions give us a better understanding of why the muscle is divided into three groups. The fibers of the upper section pull vertically, thereby raising the shoulder blade. The horizontally directed fibers of the middle section pull the shoulder blade toward the spine. The fibers of the lower section are directed almost vertically and therefore pull the shoulder blade down.

Often, an imbalance exists between the three sections. The upper fibers are often overdeveloped and very tight. This condition is due to poor prolonged posture such as forward head and rounded shoulders and repetitive daily activities in this posture—for example computer use. Because of this poor posture and overdeveloped upper fibers, the middle and lower fibers are often underdeveloped and weak. Rounded shoulders are evidence of this underdevelopment. It is crucial to address these imbalances by focusing on strengthening the mid and lower sections of the trapezius muscle in order to stabilize and brace the shoulders to attain proper posture and prevent future injuries.

## CLOSURE

Pilates addresses important aspects of a healthy musculoskeletal system, i.e., core strength, good posture and flexibility of the muscles, as well as the balance between the muscle groups. Furthermore, Pilates emphasizes strengthening the important stabilizing muscles of the musculoskeletal system, and therefore is very effective in increasing core stability. Because of this, Pilates is a great way to condition the body, to strengthen it for many athletic endeavors and to help prevent injuries.

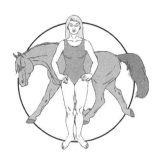

# CHAPTER 3
# GETTING STARTED

As with beginning any exercise program, it is advisable to first check with your doctor to be sure it is safe to do so.

It is tempting, when starting something new, to want to dive in with excitement and run with the new experience. However, like dressage, learning—and truly understanding—the basics of the discipline is paramount to the practice of Pilates. The basic concepts of Pilates must be understood and practiced continually so the foundation of strength and flexibility with control is solid and may be called on in challenging situations. When starting to work with the basic concepts and exercises, you will be employing the first three principles of Pilates: centering, concentration and control.

## PILATES CONCEPTS AND CONSIDERATIONS

As we have discussed, the two overarching concepts of Pilates are the "Powerhouse" and the "Box." These two concepts refer to specific areas of the body that are defined in Chapter 2 as the "core" and the "trunk." The Powerhouse and Box will be explained in this chapter in reference to the Pilates Method. Besides these two concepts, there are other important considerations that are key to making Pilates not just exercise but, rather, a new, more efficient way to use the body. It is important to take the time to understand and experiment with these considerations before you begin the Pilates exercises in

Chapter 4. By doing so, this will not only help you to avoid any soreness or injury, but it will also help you get the most out of the exercises.

Pay special attention when you see a "WHOA! TRY THIS!" or "HEADS UP!" These are especially important for the reader to help understand a concept or consideration important to Pilates, as well as for safety concerns that the reader needs to be aware of when exercising.

## THE POWERHOUSE

The Powerhouse, in essence, is a band around the midsection of the body, which includes your transversus abdominis (TA), gluteals and upper thighs. How these muscles work together to make up the major part of the body's core has been explained in Chapter 2. In Pilates, we refer to these muscles as simply the "stomach" and "bottom." Engaging these muscles deeply at all times while performing the exercises becomes the challenge for the student and is the heart of Pilates. The engagement of the Powerhouse muscles while moving is exactly the challenge we ask of the horse when we move from movement to movement, such as from piaffe to passage. If the engagement is not there, the work is not true and correct. This is the same for Pilates and is what defines Pilates as not just exercise, but also as a discipline and an art.

## IN AND UP

One of the first directives of a Pilates lesson is to "scoop the stomach in and up." This expression means to pull your abdominals, specifically the TA, in a back and upward direction toward your spine. Done correctly, this "scooping" of the abdominals will have a sensation of both a lift of the spine reaching up "through the withers and out the poll," as well as a stretch in the lower back as it lengthens the tailbone down into the saddle. Scooping the stomach in and up can also be felt as though your waistline is getting narrower in the front of the body while the back of the waistline, or lower back, feels wider.

As explained in Chapter 2, the TA is the deepest abdominal muscle (See Figure 2-4). Encircling the trunk, it provides stability to the trunk when dynamic forces would otherwise create instability. Often when one is directed to use the abdominals, it is the rectus abdominis or "six-pack" muscle that is engaged. Although this is an important core and postural muscle, it does not attach to the

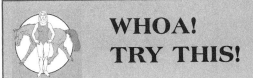

# WHOA!
# TRY THIS!

Sitting in a comfortable position, place one hand on your stomach and the other on your lower back. Now poke the belly out, expanding your waistline forward. Feel how your lower back arches and your back becomes hollow and tight.

Now in contrast, keep your hands on your stomach and lower back, and engage your TA by pulling your stomach in and up toward your spine. (If you were in a bathing suit with a photographer in the room, this is what most women would probably do!) You will want to experience this activation of your TA without tensing your shoulders or holding your breath. As you scoop your stomach in, feel your waistline very narrow in the front while your lower back feels wide. Also feel your spine elongate both up toward your neck and down toward your tailbone. This feeling of the lower back long and wide is the TA stabilizing the spine with the coactivation of the multifidi. This can be referred to as the slack being taken out of the back to create a strong but supple spine.

spine and, therefore, does not provide the same stability as the TA. When the TA is strong and engaged, it will actually function as a support belt around the spine keeping the back long, wide and stable.

Learning how to engage the TA or simply, "scoop the stomach in and up," is part of what makes Pilates an exercise method that aids in changing posture. Strengthening this core muscle to take the slack out of the back will elongate the spine. This is not to be confused with taking out the natural curves of the back. The natural curves are necessary for proper function of the spine. These curves, however, are often exaggerated due to poor posture (See Figure 2-3). Pilates serves to correct such skeletal deviations by using the Powerhouse to elongate the spine back to optimum posture (See Figure 2-2).

Because many people have some degree of the poor posture as seen in Figure 2-3, Pilates requires the practitioner to take precautions in order not to injure the

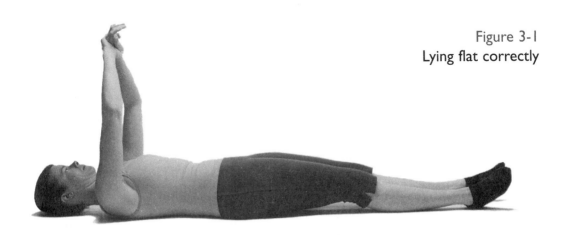

Figure 3-1
**Lying flat correctly**

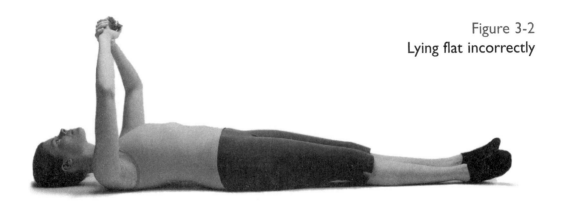

Figure 3-2
**Lying flat incorrectly**

# HEADS UP!

If you have an extreme hyperextension of the lower back or sway back, (See Figure 3-2), it will be more difficult to keep your lower back on the floor if your legs are straight. If this is the case, it is important that you keep your knees bent at all times in combination with a slight tucking under of the pelvis. This is referred to as a posterior pelvic tilt (See Figure 3-3). Ideally, one will be able to accomplish keeping the lower back touching the floor without a pelvic tilt. However, if in the beginning the lower back cannot be on the floor, it is essential to keep the knees bent and keep a slight feeling of a pelvic tilt by using the deep engagement of the Powerhouse muscles.

It is also important that you have length in your spine "through the withers and out the poll." Note in Figure 3-2 that not only is the lower back not on the floor, the neck is too arched and the rider is not "on the bit." If you cannot lengthen your neck, place a pillow under your head as seen in Figure 3-3. By doing so, not only you will be more comfortable, you will begin to stretch the muscles along the back of your neck so that is easier to be "on the bit."

Figure 3-3
Lying flat correctly with modifications

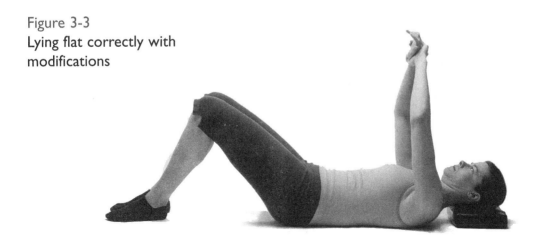

lower back. "Scooping the stomach in and up" is paramount to the safety of the Pilates practitioner. Using the stomach in this way is what will protect the lower back from discomfort and possible injury. Because most of the basic exercises are performed while lying on the back, it is essential that when you are on your back, you use the TA so the lower back can be in contact with the ground (See Figure 3-1).

# WHOA! TRY THIS!

Sitting in a chair, feel your gluteals soft and relaxed. Now squeeze the bottom. When you squeeze the bottom, you may feel a sense of slightly tucking the pelvis under and a lengthening of the lower back. If you increase this squeeze, the muscle action will help create a posterior tilt of the pelvis, which is helpful for stretching out a tight lower back. It also works with the abdominals to put the whole lower back on the ground when lying down.

As you squeeze the bottom, notice that your upper inner thighs can also engage. This feels as though the backs of your thighs are coming closer together with an outward rotating action of the hip. The movement of outward rotation in the hips can be described as the backs of the thighs "wrapping" around from the back to the front (See Figure 2-7). For the rider, this hip action is not intended to rotate the legs outward! It is used to develop stability of the seat and the ability to use the upper inner thighs to communicate "forward" to the horse.

## Squeeze the Bottom!

The second Pilates directive, simply put, is "squeeze the bottom." This refers to the engagement of the gluteals with the hip external rotators and hip adductors as explained in Chapter 2. These muscles play a supporting role in core strength. Strengthening these muscles encourages movement to be generated from the powerful muscles of the hip (haunches) rather than using the knees. Movement generated in this way can alleviate pressure on the knee joint. Also, just as good-moving horses lower their haunches for pushing power, learning to use these muscles becomes helpful for any type of body movement to be more powerful. Squeezing the bottom also will aid in creating a posterior pelvic tilt necessary for those who have an extreme sway in the lower back.

This dynamic action of the upper thighs can also be compared to that of an old-fashioned wringer washing machine, continually rotating around. Feel the inner

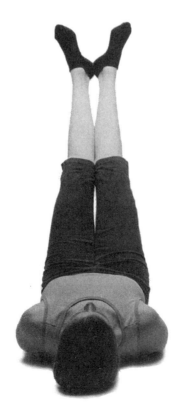

Figure 3-4
**Lying with "legs zippered"**

# HEADS UP!

Whether standing or lying down, be sure not to hyperextend, or "lock," your knees when you squeeze your bottom. This is very difficult to feel in the beginning, however, this is important for avoiding stress or pain in the knees. (Refer to Chapter 2 regarding hypermobile joints.) In all exercises that require a straight leg, it is easy to overstraighten the knee joint. Avoid this by thinking of squeezing the bottom and "zipping" the inner thighs together from the top of the leg down to just above the knee. The knee joints remain straight but "soft."

thighs "zipping" together from the top of the leg down to just above the knees as pictured in Figure 3-4. The combined muscle actions of the bottom and upper thighs create the base of support for the trunk of the body.

In Pilates this complex muscle group of gluteals and hip adductors, simplified as "squeezing of the bottom" and "wrapping the legs," creates a dynamic stance utilized in Pilates exercises performed both standing and lying down. The outward rotated hip causes the heels to come together with the toes slightly turned outwards (See Figure 2-7). If the practitioner is tight, it is advisable to ignore this stance and keep the legs together and work the exercises with bent knees. However if the practitioner has good flexibility in her hamstrings, she is encouraged to utilize this stance. The concern about working in this straight-legged stance is that a person with hypermobility in the knee will find it difficult not to "lock" the knee joint. (Refer to Chapter 2 for more information on hypermobile joints.) If this is the case, it is important that the practitioner understand how to "keep the knees soft" by experimenting with how to properly and safely engage the muscles to create this dynamic stance.

Experiment with this concept when both standing and lying down. Engage your Powerhouse and place your heels together and toes slightly apart. If you lock

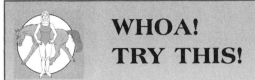

**WHOA!
TRY THIS!**

To understand hyperextension in the knee, try experimenting with the following. Sit on the floor with your legs out in front of you. Flex your ankles, reaching your toes toward the ceiling. Now, grip your quadriceps to straighten your leg. If you are hypermobile in your knees, your heels will lift up off the ground, and the backs of your knees will touch the ground (See Figure 3-5).

To have soft knees, release your quadriceps and place your heels on the ground. Pull your stomach in and squeeze your bottom. As you do this, allow your knees to straighten only to the point where your heels can stay on the floor (See Figure 3-6).

your knees it will be quite difficult to keep your heels together, and you will probably feel your lower back shorten. Now, soften the knees. You will be able to keep your heels together and feel your Powerhouse engage more deeply.

The concept of using the Pilates Powerhouse to strengthen the core and trunk is the basis of learning to use the body more efficiently. The first goal is to be able to feel a strong center to support good posture. Good posture implies not only the ability to stand up straight, but also owning the ability to use the body efficiently in any position or action of the spine. Having a strong Pilates

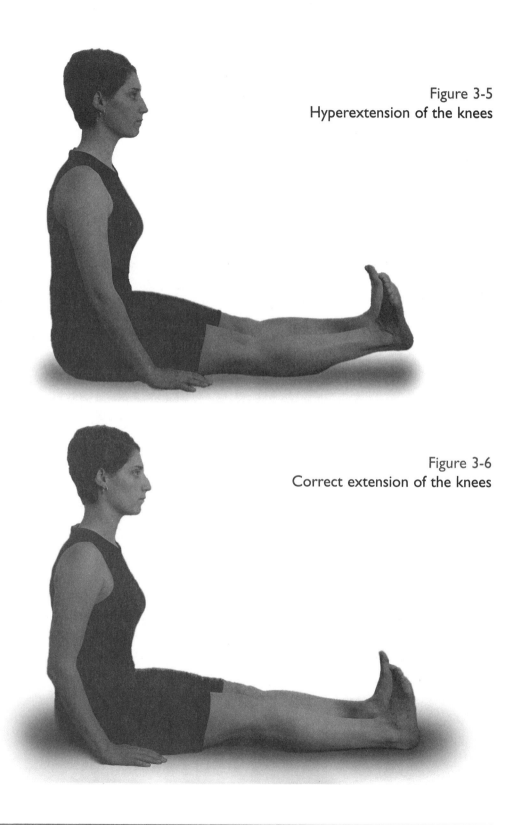

Figure 3-5
Hyperextension of the knees

Figure 3-6
Correct extension of the knees

Powerhouse gives the practitioner the ability to stay centered while allowing the neck, arms and legs to move with more freedom.

Good riding requires the ability to have independent seat, legs and hands. A core that is not adequately stabilized is evidenced when the rider grips with her legs and/or uses her hands for balance. This incorrect and inefficient use of the body inhibits the clarity of the rider's aids. The only way to have independent seat, legs and hands is to understand how to develop and maintain a strong and supple center by utilizing the muscles of the core and trunk.

# THE BOX

The second Pilates concept is to think of your trunk as a "Box" (See Figure 2-1). A proper Pilates Box requires optimum posture and symmetrical muscular development. Chapter 2 described the trunk muscles important for good posture. The specific postural muscles that Pilates develops are the mid and lower trapezius (See Figure 2-8). These muscles help keep the Box "square." The engagement of these muscles by the action of pulling shoulders "back and down" will contribute to a fully engaged spine and help to improve posture as well as symmetry in the trunk.

When looking at a properly aligned Box from the front, the right shoulder is vertically in alignment with the right hip. The left shoulder is in alignment with the left hip. The right and left shoulders are level in a horizontal line, parallel to the ground. Another horizontal, parallel line will intersect the right and left hips. When looking at the body from the side, a plumb line can be drawn from the ear, through the middle of the shoulder, ribs, hips, knee and ankle (See Figure 2-2). For the rider, this Box posture is exactly the same, except when mounted, the knee is bent (See Figure 6-1).

Often, this optimum Box symmetry that is important to riders has been compromised. Just as a horse favors one side over the other, the human body also has its asymmetries. If you observe yourself and others both on the ground and in the saddle, you will begin to notice many imbalances such as a preference to sit on one seat bone more prominently than the other; one shoulder is higher than the other; the torso rotates easily to one side and is more difficult to rotate to the other. These tendencies may be slight, but after years of these habitual movements or holding patterns, the muscles change to accommodate the tendency. One muscle becomes longer while its counterpart shortens. These muscle imbalances usually create poor posture leading to discomfort, chronic pain and, eventually, injury. Refer back to Chapter 2 for more information on muscle imbalances.

When mounted, muscle imbalances and asymmetries in the rider can contribute to poor performance of the horse. Often a rider is unable to create a shoulder-in to the right, yet, when another rider gets on the same horse, the horse magically seems to be able to do the exercise. If a rider cannot sit symmetrically on the

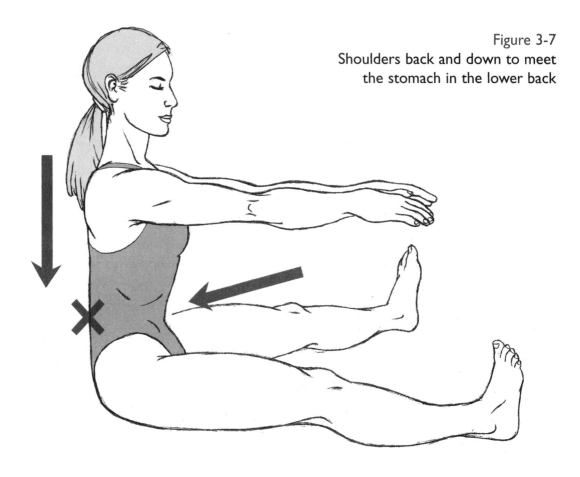

Figure 3-7
Shoulders back and down to meet
the stomach in the lower back

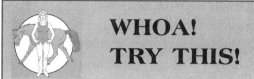

## WHOA! TRY THIS!

To feel the use of the shoulder blade muscles, try this exercise: Pinch your shoulder blades together and allow your ribs to poke out forward. Feel how this causes your back to hollow as your rib cage and chest expand forward.

Now engage the Powerhouse. Scoop the stomach in and up, squeeze the bottom, and feel the spine lengthen both up and down. Now, add the engagement of the mid and lower trapezius. To feel this, think of pulling your shoulders back and down to meet your stomach in your lower back (See Figure 3-7). You should feel your chest open and your neck elongate. When you engage these muscles, be sure your ribs do not move forward causing the back to hollow or shorten. To keep your ribs in place, feel them pull in toward each other as if they were going to be tied together. Pilates often refers to this feeling as engaging the upper abdominals.

horse, her aids become unclear. A heavier weighted right seat bone can inhibit a clear left lead canter aid. A torso with a tendency to rotate to the right can make bending a horse to the left much more difficult. Done correctly, the Pilates work will aid in correcting these muscular imbalances.

Generally, when a person begins a Pilates program (Introductory and Training Levels) the use of the mid and lower trapezius or "keeping the shoulders back and down" is not emphasized. This is because finding and engaging the Powerhouse is the essential concept for the beginner and, most often, it is not easy to concentrate on anything other than that. However, just as in First Level, the dressage horse is now asked to be on the bit while trotting a 20 meter circle, as work in Pilates progresses, engagement of the shoulder muscles back and down is preferred while performing all Pilates exercises.

For the rider, the engagement of mid and lower trapezius is essential for keeping the stability and symmetry in the whole trunk. Although the seat may be stabilized, without the use of these muscles, it will be difficult for the rider to use her arms independently. Therefore it is important for the rider to find and use the mid and lower trapezius as she begins her Pilates work.

To accommodate movement with stability, the Box must be strong but not rigid. The Powerhouse and Box muscles must be able to minutely adjust to compensate for movement in the legs and arms and the dynamic force of the horse's back on the rider's seat. The practice of Pilates will teach the rider to be able to command the right amount of muscle engagement necessary to keep the core and trunk lengthened and dynamically engaged. Having these abilities will give the rider the true freedom to have an independent seat, legs and hands.

# A WORD ABOUT BREATHING

There are specific breathing patterns to every Pilates exercise. As you move up the Pilates training scale, rhythm, flow, and breath are the more advanced principles. Each exercise has a breath rhythm designed to help the movement flow. However, in the beginning, executing the exercises with proper attention to the Powerhouse and Box is enough to think about. Therefore the Pilates practitioner should mainly focus on not holding the breath. Usually one will manage to take in a breath but, often, due to tension or concentration on a particular movement, the breath is held. The emphasis in the beginning, then, is to ensure the practitioner does not hold her breath while performing the exercises. Only after the exercises are fairly familiar should the breathing patterns be attempted.

When the practitioner begins to focus on the breathing patterns, she may find that it is very different from breathing patterns taught in most other exercise regimens. If the use of the breath is not understood, the practitioner should seek a qualified Pilates instructor to help her understand how to properly breathe so

## WHOA!
## TRY THIS!

Place your hands on your stomach and a take a deep breath. When you inhale, you will feel the abdominal wall expand. When you exhale the abdominal wall will relax down. This is how you normally breathe. Now hold the abdominal wall back (pull the stomach in and up) and take in a deep breath. Exhale and pull the stomach in more. Inhale again keeping the stomach in. This is the essence of using the breath to help strengthen the TA.

When you begin the first Pilates exercise—the Hundreds—you will experience this challenge. Each breath you take will challenge the TA to remain engaged, pulling back toward the spine. When you exhale, press the abdominal wall farther back and keep it there as the next breath comes in.

that the exercises can be performed safely. Pilates work teaches the practitioner to actively pull the stomach in and up whether she is inhaling or exhaling. It is relatively easy to pull the stomach in while exhaling. To keep the abdominals in while inhaling can be more difficult. As the air is taken in, it will naturally expand the abdominal wall. Pulling the stomach in against this force requires the TA to work even harder. This serves to strengthen the TA more efficiently than other forms of abdominal exercising. Although difficult to do, when this is mastered the practitioner gains control over the deepest core muscle. This gives the rider the ability to utilize this important core stabilizing muscle while executing movements over a period of time when it is essential to breathe continually.

At first, it may feel impossible to breathe when the stomach is in and up. If this is the case, there are several ways to think about taking in a breath. Normal breathing is often referred to as diaphragmatic breathing. This is what is felt when the abdominal wall expands. However since the lungs are three dimensional, one can direct the breath into the upper chest or the back with a feeling of the back expanding. One can also direct the breath sideways. This feels like the back of the rib cage widens side to side under the arms. You will want to experiment with sending the breath in different directions to find a way that works for you.

# THE ENGAGEMENT OF THE HUMAN SPINE

To perform dressage correctly, your horse must be relaxed and supple, engaged and travel within a circle of energy, which begins from the horses hind legs, moves up over the back, up the neck and out the poll to be recycled into the rider's hands. From this engagement comes the ability to supple the horse longitudinally and hence, the ability to lengthen and collect the horse for the movements required as the horse moves up the levels. How many times have you heard this and other statements like it? And how many times have you been puzzled during lessons when your instructor was calling out one correction after the other with terms such as "half halt," "rounder" or "allow him to lengthen more," but never offered how to do these things in a way that was easily accomplished?

As a rider moves up the levels, she cannot deny that these concepts become essential. But understanding them, feeling them and being able to use aids to create this energy in the horse are quite the mystery for most dressage riders. By First Level, the rider already needs to know how to lengthen a horse's stride in trot and canter. By Second Level, the rider needs to know how to collect the walk, trot and canter as well as to lengthen them. Beyond that, riders need to be able to keep a horse supple and relaxed while completely engaged in order to correctly perform movements and transitions between movements. It is no wonder, then, that in most dressage shows the numbers of competitors begins to quickly diminish after Training Level.

Understanding how to use the Pilates Powerhouse will give you the experience of having control over—or what is termed in dressage as "engagement of"—the spine. Most riders know the feeling when the horse is not engaged and there is no circle of energy. The horse becomes disconnected, drops his back and tenses his neck. Often the rider, too, becomes disengaged without knowing it. She hollows her back, stiffens her neck and braces herself with her arms and legs for balance. If the rider had the ability to lengthen and collect her own spine, she probably would have a better understanding of engagement of the horse's spine. Not only that, by keeping herself engaged, she will inevitably develop the ability to keep her horse engaged.

# UNDERSTANDING ENGAGEMENT

For the purposes of this book, engagement can be defined as the ability to have active muscular control over both the strength and flexibility of the muscles of the body in order to use all parts of the body at will and with precision. It is beyond the scope of this book to anatomically detail how the horse actually uses his musculature for engagement during movement. The discussion that follows generalizes the concepts to help the reader/rider understand the basis of what is required of the dressage horse so she may begin to feel the same concept in her own spine.

Using Pilates exercises to balance flexibility with strength in the core and trunk will help create engagement in the rider. As explained in Chapter 2, too much flexibility in the spine or lack of suppleness, can lead to instability for the rider. Having the ability to control, or engage, a strong and supple core will allow the rider to use her body more efficiently. With this control over the body comes the ability to communicate clearer and more precise aids to the horse. Also, if the rider can understand and feel engagement in her own spine, she may more quickly detect and be able to respond to the engagement—or lack thereof—in her horse.

Both Pilates and dressage demand engagement from the practitioner and the horse so they can fully use their flexibility with control. In order to achieve this, the rider and horse must work to not only have optimal flexibility but also to develop maximum muscle strength through exercises designed to integrate and balance both in order to achieve control over movement. The rider attempting a shoulder-in must have control over—be engaged—in her core and trunk. If she is stiff in her core, she is not able to finely tune the rotation in her spine needed to help the horse execute an accurate shoulder-in. If she is too flexible, she does not have the strength to hold her body in a strong, yet supple position to maintain the horse in the movement.

# CREATING FLEXIBILITY IN THE CORE AND TRUNK

### DEEP AND ROUND

Referring to the postural deviations described in Chapter 2, it becomes apparent that attention to the spinal and pelvic muscles is indicated for most people. Often people think of flexibility in terms of hamstring or calf muscles. Although flexibility in these muscle groups is important, postural deviations are most often caused by shortened and weak muscles in the hips, lower back and neck. Since the spine is at the core of the rider's seat and the horse's athletic abilities, stretching the spine is usually the first goal for both the horse and rider.

Figure 3-8
Horse stretching deep and round

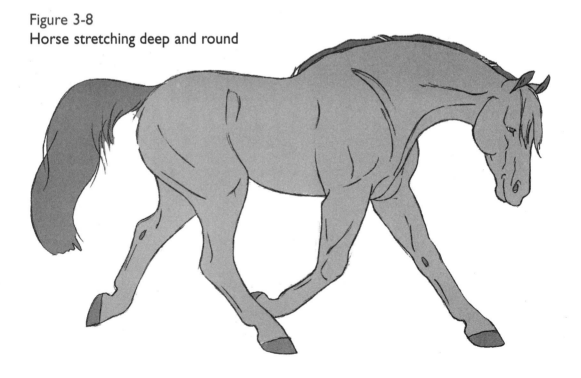

This stretching is not done passively. Rather, dynamic stretching of the spine for both horse and rider requires the use of the Pilates Powerhouse.

To create flexibility in the spine of a horse, exercises are often given that are referred to as "long and low" or "deep and round" (see Figure 3-8). The ultimate goal of these exercises is that, executed correctly, the horse will attain the maximum stretch in his spine, or top-line, by using the maximum contraction of his underside muscles. Simplifying this complex muscular action of how a horse collects his spine into Pilates vocabulary can help the reader/rider begin to identify how her body can do the same. As the horse scoops his stomach in and up and engages his bottom muscles, he shortens the underside of his body creating a dynamic stretch over his entire back. This stretch affects a rounded back posture, allowing the horse's pelvis to "sit down" and use his bottom muscles. The hind legs are then able to step underneath his body creating an even more dynamic stretch in his spine. His abdominals are encouraged to push the back upward, making the spine round and supple. Through this engaged, yet supple spine, the energy generated by the horse's haunches can move over his back and into his neck and poll. This traveling of energy is often termed "throughness." Developing this dynamic stretch or throughness in the back will

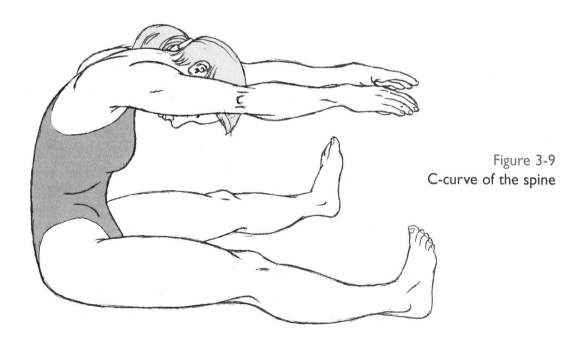

Figure 3-9
C-curve of the spine

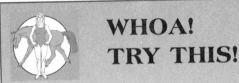

# WHOA! TRY THIS!

Get down on your hands and knees. Arch your back and lift your chin like a hollowed out horse. Keeping this back position, "step" forward with a "hind leg." Notice how far you can step forward.

Now, engage your Powerhouse. Scoop your abdominals into your spine and squeeze your gluteals to elongate your lower back, sit your pelvis down and round your spine, making the shape of the letter "C". Feel your stomach pushing the ribs back toward the spine—think round and deep. Again, step forward with your hind leg. You will find that you can step much farther underneath yourself.

allow the horse to rely on the power of the center of his body so he can relax his neck in order to move his whole body with more freedom.

Pilates creates a deep-and-round stretch for the human in the same way. It is referred to as the C-curve of the spine, meaning the spine creates the shape of the letter "C" (see Figure 3-9). This stretch is accomplished by using the Pilates Powerhouse. When the stomach is in and up and the bottom is engaged, the front of the body contracts maximally so the back can fully stretch. This stretch, especially through the lower back, allows the pelvis to "sit" down, which anchors the stretch. The abdominals then can be used to push the rib cage back toward the spine to stretch—or round—the back. The use of the Powerhouse stabilizes the center of the body so the energy of the stretch continues up to the "withers" (back of the neck), and the neck becomes free to be "on the bit." This dynamic stretch or C-curve of the spine strengthens the Pilates Powerhouse. With this strength and flexibility, the practitioner will have the tools to understand and achieve engagement to lengthen and collect her own spine.

# Lengthening and Collecting the Spine

Working toward flexibility in the spine by strengthening the abdominals and gluteals is the first step to achieving engagement. Now the horse and rider must develop the control over this strength and flexibility in order to use the length of the back for both collected and extended gaits. The control over elongated musculature is key to staying engaged during lengthening.

For the horse to properly extend or collect his gaits, he must control his spine with the use of his Powerhouse muscles. As described in the preceding discussion, to stretch, round or collect the spine, the horse must pull his stomach muscles in and up while his bottom muscles engage so he can "sit" or anchor his pelvis. This anchoring of the pelvis allows his back to stretch while enabling him to swing his hind legs forward to step up well underneath his body. The stepping through allows him to round his back even more, so the energy of the stretch can move through his back to free his neck and poll.

To remain engaged while lengthening, the horse must keep his Powerhouse muscles actively engaged, releasing them only as needed to elongate his spine. This active muscular use of his "Powerhouse" muscles keeps his back round or engaged while his spine is allowed to elongate. The stabilized power from behind and center allows the horse to freely move forward, lengthening his spine with no undue tension in his shoulders, neck and poll.

While lengthening or collecting, if the abdominal muscles are not kept engaged, the horse's back becomes hollow and the neck tenses and shortens. The haunches become disengaged as the pelvis lifts up and back instead of scooping down and forward. With the spine in this inverted shape, the horse's hind legs cannot possibly reach up underneath his body. Therefore the horse cannot truly collect or lengthen his stride because his spine is not engaged.

In the same way, the human spine can, with the use of the Powerhouse muscles, lengthen and collect. When the practitioner wants to stretch out her spine maximally, doing so dynamically, she will actually collect her spine. Using the bottom to anchor the stretch, the abdominal muscles push in and up to achieve a rounded back, allowing the head and neck muscles to release tension. This dynamically rounded back can be perceived as collection.

With control, the practitioner can lengthen her spine from this strong center. Having the stabilized power in the bottom and center allows for the release of tension in the shoulders, neck and head. From this deeply rounded position of the spine, she can move to a straighter but engaged spine by releasing the Powerhouse muscles only as needed to create a straighter (or lengthened) spine.

If not elongated with the use of the Powerhouse muscles, the back of the human or horse will actually shorten, hollow and the chin will lift causing the neck to become short and tense. This is not an efficient use of the body. For the horse, this posture is termed in many ways: the horse "is not working over his back," "not on the bit," "not engaged." This improper way of going cannot further the horse's dressage capabilities (see Figure 3-10).

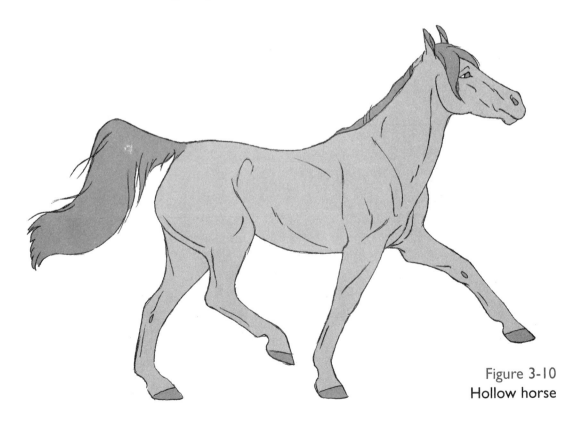

Figure 3-10
**Hollow horse**

For the rider, this inefficient use of musculature will affect her riding abilities. Her lower back will shorten through excess tension and allow her stomach to stretch out. This causes an anterior tilt (swayback) of the pelvis and the rider has no driving seat. The neck also will shorten and create a forward head. This poor posture does not allow the rider to have a balanced seat, which means she will use her arms and legs to balance and, therefore, her aids will be inhibited (see Figure 3-11).

Elongating the natural curves of the spine by using the Pilates Powerhouse creates a deeper and more balanced seat. It allows the spine to remain supple and lengthened while remaining engaged.

The ability to use the Powerhouse muscles to control the collection and lengthening of the spine at will is necessary for both the Pilates practitioner and the dressage horse. Many of the Pilates exercises will give the rider the sense of how the horse remains engaged while elongating the spine from collection to

Figure 3-11
**Hollow human**

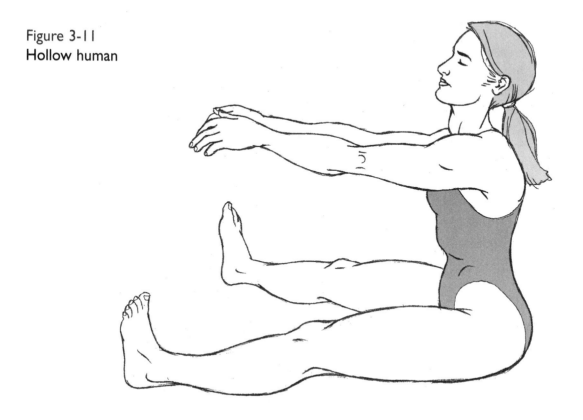

Get down on your hands and knees. Engage your Powerhouse: Pull your abdominals in and up and squeeze your gluteals to elongate the lower back and round your spine. Feel your stomach pushing your ribs back toward the spine and think "C-curve" or "round and deep." You are now "collected."

Now release your Powerhouse muscles completely! Feel how this total release of the Powerhouse sways your lower back and lifts your chin. This full release of the Powerhouse muscles does not lengthen the back. Notice how the lower back and neck have been allowed to shorten with undue tension in the muscles. This is the feeling of "lengthening" the spine without engagement.

Return to the deep and round position. Using your Powerhouse muscles with control, slowly lengthen your spine. By remaining dynamically engaged as you perform this movement, you will achieve the feeling of a true lengthening of the spine.

extension. The reader/rider is encouraged to continue the exploration of using the developing Powerhouse muscles to deepen the understanding of engagement in her own spine. Without engagement, the spine is at the mercy of motion and cannot be the center through which all movement is controlled. Keeping engagement in both the horse and the human spine is the essence of moving with power and grace.

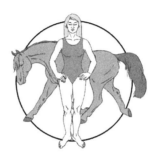

# CHAPTER 4
# BASIC PILATES MAT WORKOUT

The basic Pilates exercises are important to the Dressage rider for many reasons. First, they will establish the concepts of the Pilates Powerhouse and the Pilates Box, which leads to a better understanding of supporting proper posture and symmetry in the body. Second, they serve as a warm-up before mounting. Third, they become a basis for the exercises in Chapter 5, "Advancing Pilates Exercises" and Chapter 6, "Mounted Pilates Exercises." Honing these basic exercises helps the reader/rider feel the engagement of the human spine, through which the rider will develop a greater understanding of the same in the horse's spine. The final goal is to find, using these basic exercises, a practical understanding of how Pilates exercises and concepts can make you a better rider, which is addressed specifically in Chapter 7.

As with beginning any exercise program, it is advisable to first check with your doctor to be sure it is safe to do so. When you perform the following exercises, it is good if you feel your abdominal and gluteal muscles getting warm from the work. You also might feel stretching of your hamstrings and upper back. It is essential, however, that there is no discomfort in the neck or lower back. If you do have any discomfort, seek professional help immediately. If you feel discomfort in any other part of the body, consult Chapter 3 again. If you still cannot relieve the discomfort, consult a Pilates instructor, your doctor or physical therapist to be sure you are performing the exercises correctly. You should perform these exercises on a firm mat or on carpet to pad and protect the spine.

Remember the cautions in Chapter 3. If your chin lifts up to the ceiling when you are lying down you may want a small pillow for under your head. If you need to, do not hesitate to bend your knees so your lower back is always in contact with the floor when you are lying down.

In all exercises, the use of the Pilates Powerhouse is emphasized. What is not specifically mentioned is the fact that, in all exercises, close attention should be paid to the symmetry of the Pilates Box. The "squareness" of the Box is implied by use of Powerhouse muscles and the shoulders being pulled back and down by the mid and lower trapezius. It is important to note that although you may feel that you are working correctly, you may have some asymmetries in your Box. To correct this, you may want to work with a mirror or a partner to check that the Box remains square and symmetrical at all times.

# HUNDREDS

This exercise will stimulate the lungs to work deeply and help the blood begin to circulate through the body to warm up your muscles. Think of it as the first trot of the ride, on the bit, engaged and lively.

## STEP ONE
Lie on your back and bend your knees into your chest. Pull your stomach in and up to anchor your lower back to the floor. Be sure there is no space between your low back and the floor or mat. Elongate your arms by your sides by pulling your shoulders down to meet your stomach in your lower back. If you can do so without your neck hurting, bring your chin up toward your chest.

## STEP TWO
Extend your legs toward the ceiling. If the backs of your legs are tight, keep your knees slightly bent and parallel to each other. If you can maintain your low back on the floor, extend your legs straight and squeeze your bottom so your hips rotate outward bringing your heels together and your toes apart. Your upper thighs should feel like an old-fashioned wringer washing machine—squeezing together and continually wrapping around and around (See Figure 2-7).

## STEP THREE

Begin pumping your arms up and down from your shoulder, about 4 to 6 inches. As you do this, inhale for five pumps, and exhale on the next five pumps. Keep your abdominals pulling in and up as you inhale and pull them in and up more as you exhale. Continue to feel your lower back anchored to the floor. Repeat for a total of 100 counts.

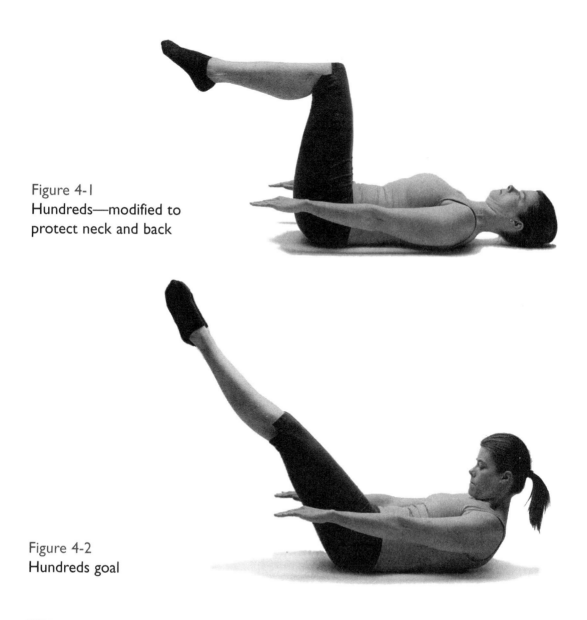

Figure 4-1
**Hundreds—modified to protect neck and back**

Figure 4-2
**Hundreds goal**

## NOTES AND GOALS

♦ Be sure your lower back stays on the ground.

♦ In general, if you need a pillow under your head at this point, you will want to do this exercise and all subsequent exercises that require the head to be up, with your head down and on the pillow.

♦ Only lift your head for a few counts at a time until you can leave your head up without any discomfort in your neck.

♦ If you feel your thighs working too hard, you will need to bend your knees until you acquire more hamstring flexibility.

♦ If you are able to extend your legs, be sure your knees are soft. Feel your thighs "zippered up" from the back of the hips to just above the knee (Refer to Figure 3-4).

♦ Your stomach should not bulge or push upward. It should be pulling down toward the floor. If you cannot pull your stomach down, try keeping your head down and bending your knees even farther toward your chest.

♦ Be sure not to reach your arms from your elbows. Instead, feel your arms reaching from your shoulder blades actively pulling back and down to meet your stomach in your lower back.

# ROLLING BACK

The purpose of this exercise is to increase the flexibility in your spine by use of the C-curve. Think of this as the ultimate engagement for deep and round.

## STEP ONE

Sit on the floor with your knees bent and your feet flat on the floor. Hold on to the underside of your thighs with both hands. Your arms will be bent, and you will use them to help you as you begin to move. Curl your chin to your chest as if you were trying to put the top of your head on your knees. Scoop your tailbone under as you pull your stomach in and up and squeeze your bottom. (This is C-curve, or the deep-and-round part of the exercise.)

## STEP TWO

Keeping the Powerhouse engaged, inhale as you begin to lower your spine toward the floor, one vertebrae at a time. This is the essence of lengthening the spine while staying engaged. Hold onto your thighs with your hands, but allow your elbows to slowly straighten to let the spine move toward the floor. Keep your chin on your chest to anchor the top part of this stretch. Go only as far as you can keep the abdominals "in and up." Hold this position for a moment while you exhale and deepen the scoop of the stomach and bottom.

## STEP THREE

To come back up, engage the Powerhouse muscles even more and, using your arms, if necessary, to help curl back up one vertebrae at a time as you inhale and return to the starting position. Exhale and release the muscles. Repeat 5-8 times.

## NOTES AND GOALS

♦ Your first goal should be to touch the back of your waistline to the floor.
♦ If your abs begin to pooch out, you have gone too low and lost engagement of your Powerhouse muscles.
♦ You can perform this exercise imagining that you are a large area rug that has been rolled up. As you unroll the carpet, it touches the floor. As you roll it back up, you want to roll it up tightly!

Figure 4-3
**Rolling Back**

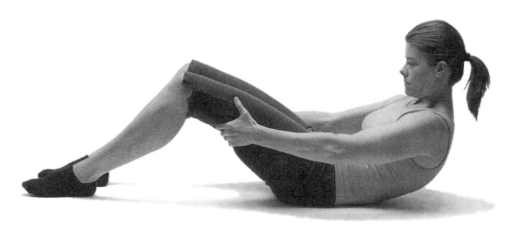

When the above exercise gets fairly easy, you may try the next exercise: the Roll Up. The Roll Up further challenges your control over the engagement of the abdominals while the spine "lengthens and collects." Your goal is to articulate the spine by "peeling" it off the floor, one vertebrae at a time and then replacing it, vertebrae by vertebrae, back down to the floor. Imagine your body as a rug being rolled up tightly, then unrolled back.

# ROLL UP

Done correctly, this is the essence of true engagement of the human spine. In this exercise you will begin with a lengthened spine, move toward collection and then back to a lengthening.

## TO GET INTO POSITION
Begin with the Rolling Back. When your waistline is on the floor, continue lowering your spine down to the floor, one vertebrae at a time. Your head will be the last part of the spine to touch. In the beginning, keep your knees bent to be sure the whole spine is touching the floor.

## STEP ONE
Lying flat on the floor, slowly reach your arms back behind your head toward the floor. Keep your arms straight, shoulder-width apart. Your ribs will want to pop up toward the ceiling and your back will try to hollow. Resist this by using the Powerhouse to keep your lower back on the ground. Your arms will probably not touch the floor. This is fine.

## STEP TWO
To begin the Roll Up, lift your arms to the ceiling and lift your head. Start to "peel" your spine off the floor by reaching your arms toward your feet. Pull your stomach in and up and squeeze your bottom to feel your lower back press into the floor as your head and upper back begin to peel off the floor. If you need help getting up, use your arms by holding the backs of your thighs with your hands and bending your elbows. Be sure you do not let your stomach pooch out.

## STEP THREE

Continue past the Rolling Back starting position and allow your legs to extend straight in front of you. Curve your spine forward so the top of your head and arms are reaching toward your feet. If you are extremely flexible, be sure when you reach that you don't collapse on top of your legs. Rather, keep your stomach lifted as if you were continuing to pull your stomach into your lower back as you reach forward.

## STEP FOUR

Bend your knees again and return your spine to the floor, passing through the Rolling Back exercise. After five or six repetitions, you will finish the exercise with your spine fully on the floor.

### NOTES AND GOALS

♦ If your stomach pooches out while performing this exercise, you will need to spend more time with the Rolling Back exercise before attempting this again.

♦ At first, focus on not holding your breath. When you are comfortable, you can inhale on the way up, exhale as you stretch over your legs, inhale as you roll down and exhale as your lift your arms back over your head.

Figure 4-4
End point of the Roll Up

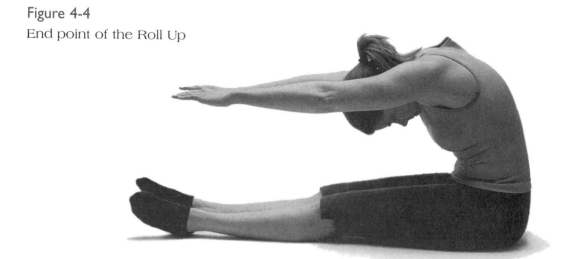

♦ When you can do this well, try to straighten your legs on both the way up and down. Most people find that having bent knees on the way up and straight knees on the way down is the first step to practice before trying the whole exercise with their legs straight.

♦ When you Roll Up, it is hard to feel your shoulders down into the lower back. However, try to feel your shoulders pulling down as you return your spine vertebrae by vertebrae to the floor. As you get stronger, try to keep your shoulders down on the way up.

# LEG CIRCLES

This exercise develops an independent seat and legs. Think of the concept of keeping your horse engaged during a leg yield.

## STEP ONE
Lie on the floor, knees bent with your feet flat on the floor. Pull your stomach in and up, and anchor your lower back on the floor. If you find your chin lifting up during the exercise try to elongate your neck by lowering your chin, or place a book or firm pillow under your head. Pull your shoulders back and down and have the sense of pulling your shoulders down to meet your stomach in your lower back as you reach down toward your feet with your arms and palms on the floor at your sides.

## STEP TWO
With a soft knee, lift up your right leg to the ceiling. If you are tight, keep your knee bent. Take a hold of the lifted leg with both hands and gently stretch it toward you. Hold the leg either above or below the knee, being sure not to hold the knee joint itself.

## STEP THREE
Leave your right leg extended as much as possible toward the ceiling and return your arms to your sides. With your heel turned inward in line with the center of your body and your toe angling out to the side, make a circle with your leg the size of a volleyball. Inhale as you cross your leg over the centerline of the body just as a horse steps up underneath himself during a leg yield.

Continue the circle of your leg down and then around away from the centerline of your body. (This part of the movement would be pushing away step of the leg yield.) Exhale as your leg finishes the circle with your heel in line with the center of your body, back at the starting position. Repeat 5 times and then reverse the direction of the circle. Repeat the exercise with your left leg.

## NOTES AND GOALS

♦ Keep your lower back firmly anchored to the floor. If you feel the hips rocking from side to side while performing the circle of the leg, pull in your stomach more and reduce the size of the circles.

♦ Feel the movement of the leg being initiated from your hip.

♦ If your hamstrings are tight, keep the knee of the leg that is circling bent as well as the leg that is on the ground.

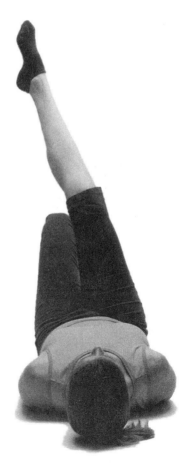

Figure 4-5
**Leg Circles**

♦ Crossing of the centerline of your body (stepping underneath yourself) while being completely engaged in the abdominals is the most important part of the exercise. You should feel the stretch on the outside of your hip and thigh.

♦ As your leg travels away from your body, be sure the opposite hip remains anchored to the floor. Engage the bottom of this leg to help stabilize your hips.

♦ Work toward eventually having both legs straight.

# SINGLE LEG STRETCH

This exercise strengthens the Powerhouse muscles and creates flexibility in your hips, legs and lower back. Think of this as an extended trot. Your thighs will be stretching and reaching away from each other just as a horse's front leg needs to reach forward from the shoulder as the back leg is pushing off. You will do this while remaining engaged in your core.

## STEP ONE

Lie on your back. Engage your abdominals in and up with your lower back anchored on the floor. Bend your knees to your chest. Place your right hand on your right ankle and your left hand just below your right knee. (If you have knee problems, you can place both hands on the back of your thigh.) Hug your right knee to your chest. This particular hand position is designed to align your hip, knee and ankle. While hugging your right knee to your chest, elongate your left leg from your hip. To do this, keep your knee soft and feel the gluteus of the left leg engage (the "pushing-off" muscle), and rotate your hip outward like a single-legged "wringer washing machine."

## STEP TWO

If you can, lift your chin to your chest. Keeping your abdominals engaged, change legs, now hugging your left knee to your chest with the left hand on the left ankle and the right hand just below your knee. Your right leg will reach long from your hip by engaging the right gluteus. Repeat this eight times for each leg.

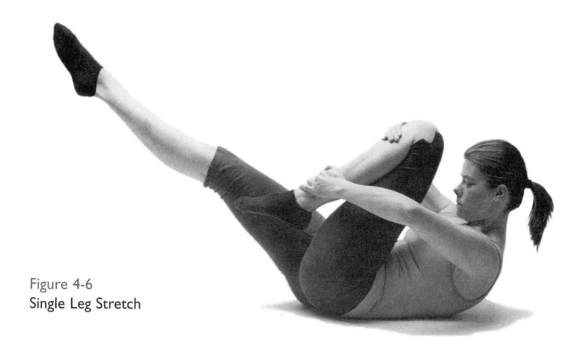

Figure 4-6
**Single Leg Stretch**

## NOTES AND GOALS

♦ Keep your abdominals engaged deeply as you change legs.

♦ If your neck gets tired, put your head down as needed.

♦ Feel your shoulders pulling down into the back of your waist while your elbows lift to feel a wide stretch across the back of your shoulders and neck.

♦ The breathing pattern of this exercise will change depending on the tempo. In the beginning, take the exercise slowly, inhaling while you bring your right knee to your chest, and exhaling when you bring your left knee to your chest.

♦ Remember that the hand position is designed to align the ankle, knee and hip joints. If you have knee problems, be sure to hold the thigh under the knee to avoid pressure on your knee joint.

# DOUBLE LEG STRETCH

In the beginning, this exercise is essentially performed as a collected movement only. The difference between this and some of the other deep-and-round
or C-curve exercises is that it requires you to collect while lying on your back.
The force of gravity on your arms and legs while lying on your back challenges
the engagement of your Powerhouse as you gradually begin to lengthen the
spine. The ultimate goal of this exercise is a full lengthening and collection of
your spine.

## STEP ONE

Lie on your back and hug both knees to your chest. Your hands can hold your
legs to your chest on top of your ankles or under your thighs if you have knee
problems. It is important that, in this exercise, you lift your chin to your chest. If
you cannot lift your head, you should avoid straightening your legs (see Figure
4-7). Engage your Powerhouse and feel your spine lengthen with your lower
back anchored into the floor.

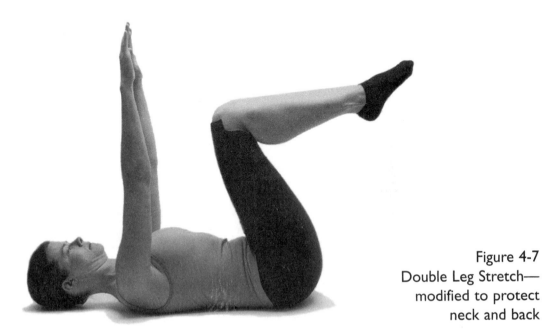

Figure 4-7
Double Leg Stretch—
modified to protect
neck and back

## STEP TWO

Keeping your spine touching the floor with your abdominals, extend your arms and legs toward the ceiling as you inhale. You are creating a C-curve of your spine with C lying on its back. Reaching your arms and legs toward the ceiling with your chin on your chest will ensure that your lower back remains on the floor. If you are flexible enough, your legs can be straight with your bottom engaged, heels together and toes apart with the feeling of zipping and wrapping the legs.

## STEP THREE

Keeping your Powerhouse engaged, reach your arms to the side and exhale as you return your legs to your chest, hugging them with your arms.
Repeat this up to eight times.

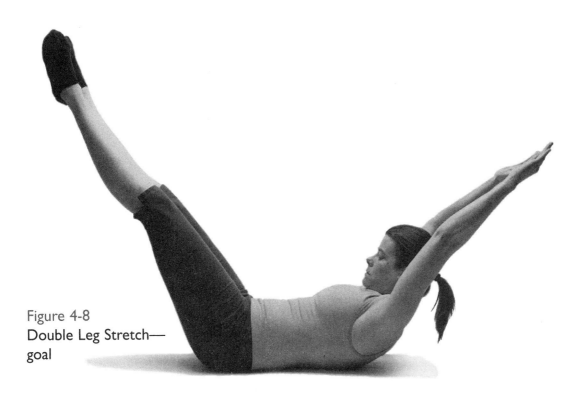

Figure 4-8
Double Leg Stretch—
goal

# HEADS UP!

It is essential to have your lower back on the floor while executing this exercise. Lifting your head to your chest helps keep the back round. If your neck gets tired, put it down, but you may need to keep your legs lifted higher or your knees bent to keep your lower back touching the floor. If you feel any discomfort in your lower back, stop immediately. It means that you are not strong enough to do this exercise correctly.

## NOTES AND GOALS

♦ As you strengthen this collected action of the spine, you may begin to use your Powerhouse strength to lengthen your spine little by little by allowing your legs to lower and straighten more. Always be sure your lower back is pressed to the floor at all times using your abdominals (See Figure 4-8). If not, you are working past your level for safe exercising.

♦ Your ultimate goal (FEI Pilates!) is to have your arms one inch off the floor behind you and your legs one inch off the floor in front of you with only your chin on your chest with your lower back on the floor and your Powerhouse fully engaged. This extension of the spine with the Powerhouse fully engaged may take years to master, so work slowly toward this goal.

# SPINE STRETCH FORWARD

This exercise is a dynamic stretch of the spine, creating suppleness in the back. As with the Rolling Back and Roll Up, this exercise will help the rider understand how to lengthen and collect her spine. This exercise begins with a lengthened spine and moves toward collection. This is also a deep breathing exercise.

## Step One

Sit with your legs out in front of you about three feet apart. If you are tight, keep your knees bent. Flex your ankles but be sure your heels are on the floor if your legs are straight (See Figures 3-5 and 3-6). Your arms will be parallel with the floor in line with your shoulders. Feel your whole back lengthened with the light engagement of your stomach, and a sense of your ribs moving back, as if you were trying to press your whole back against a wall. Your shoulder blades will pull down as if to meet your stomach in your lower back (See Figure 3-7).

## Step Two

Inhaling, squeeze your bottom and pull your stomach in and up. You want to feel your whole spine lengthen from the tailbone stretching down, up through the back of your neck and out the top of your head. Keeping your shoulders down into your back, place your chin on your chest and begin to exhale as you aim the crown of your head toward the floor between your knees. Feel as though you are peeling your spine off the wall one vertebrae at a time. Keep stretching toward the floor as you exhale deeply, feeling your stomach pulling in even more. This position is very much like the first part of the Rolling Back—deep and round.

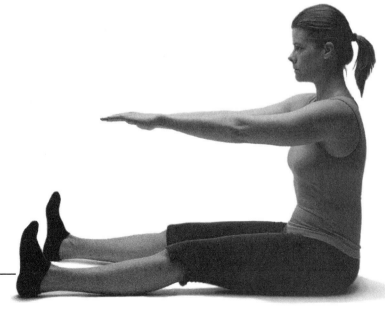

Figure 4-9
**Spine Stretch Forward—
beginning position**

## STEP THREE

Reverse the process. Inhale and roll back up through the spine. Feel as if you are placing your spine back on the wall, vertebrae by vertebrae. This involves the use of your stomach, in and up, to place your ribs in line with your hips. Feel your shoulder blades pull down into your back as you unfold your spine, bringing your head up at the last moment. Repeat 5-8 times.

## NOTES AND GOALS

♦ This is a breathing exercise. Utilize your abdominals to press the air out of your lungs, deepening the stretch in your back.

♦ On the way back up, imagine that you are "stacking" your spine, vertebrae by vertebrae, on top of each other. Your ribs will want to poke forward. Resist this, and pull them in toward each other to feel a wide and supple back.

♦ When you are in the "collected" position, you may grab your ankles and use your arms to assist in the Spine Stretch Forward.

♦ Although you may feel this in your hamstrings, the purpose is to stretch your spine!

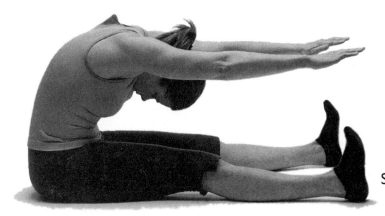

Figure 4-10
Spine Stretch Forward—
end position

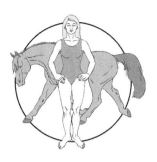

# CHAPTER 5
# ADVANCING PILATES EXERCISES

As the basic Pilates exercises become easier, you will want to advance into more challenging exercises. The basic exercises described in Chapter 4 have introduced work to build a Pilates Powerhouse and Box. In essence, this work gives the practitioner the first experience of core stability while moving. In the basic exercises, most of the movement has been performed while lying down or sitting. However as Pilates exercises develop, you will be asked to use the Powerhouse and keep the symmetry of the Box while doing exercises standing up, lying on the stomach or even, eventually, while in a push-up position on one arm. It is beyond the scope of this book to include all the beginning, inter-mediate and advanced exercises that make up the Pilates Method. Culled from more than 500 exercises that Joseph Pilates created, these next Pilates exercis-es are specifically chosen for the dressage rider to further challenge the basics while executing them in differing body positions.

The following exercises are performed not only lying down, but also while standing, lying on your stomach or on your side. Gravity will have a differing effect on the Box and will require the Powerhouse muscles to work more dynamically. In order to accomplish these more difficult exercises safely, you must perform them with precision. Your Pilates Powerhouse must be under complete control so you can maintain the stomach in and up to keep a length-ened spine before, during and after the exercise. Just as in dressage, these exercises may appear simple, but the engagement required to do them correct-ly makes them as challenging as performing a half pass as opposed to a leg yield.

## HEADS UP!

If you feel any discomfort in your lower back while performing the exercises on your stomach or on your side, stop immediately and do not attempt the exercise until you consult your Pilates instructor, doctor or physical therapist.

As in the exercises in Chapter 4, the Powerhouse and shoulder muscles are specifically discussed. What is not discussed is the overarching concept of the Box. Be sure to be mindful of its symmetry by using a mirror or friend to help you stay "square."

## OPEN LEG ROCKER POSITION (INTERMEDIATE)

This exercise works on strength and stretch with control. The postural essence of this exercise informs the basic dressage seat (See Chapter 7).

### STEP ONE

Sit on the floor with your knees bent and the soles of your feet together. Your knees will open to the sides, but only allow them to open in line with your shoulders. Holding your ankles, feel your stomach move in and up and your bottom squeeze to scoop and feel your lower back lengthen. Keep your shoulders back and down as you lift your chest and allow the back of your neck to elongate (lifting the withers). This solid position of the trunk is the engagement of the muscles of the Pilates Box and promotes your basic functional dressage seat.

### STEP TWO

Pick your feet up off the ground and balance. Your knees will be in line with your shoulders. You may feel your lower back try to help you balance by arching or pushing forward (hollow back). Be sure this does not happen by being vigilant that the stomach remains in and up and that you feel the gluteals engaged and your tail bone "scooping" so that your lower back stays long or even slightly rounded.

## STEP THREE

Slowly and carefully, begin to straighten your legs. When your legs are straight, your feet will be shoulder width apart. Keep the sense of wrapping your thighs so that your heels will be toward the center of the body and your toes will reach away from the center. As you extend your legs, keep your lower back long or slightly rounded with the engagement of the Powerhouse. Keep the chest lifted but do not allow your ribs to poke forward. Feel the withers, or the back of the base of your neck lifting. Extend your legs as far as you can, but allow your knees to remain slightly bent if you are tight, rather than compromising your body position. While balancing, feel your shoulder blades moving down toward your waistline. Inhale as you move to this extended leg position.

## STEP FOUR

Exhale as you return to the first balanced position. Repeat five times.

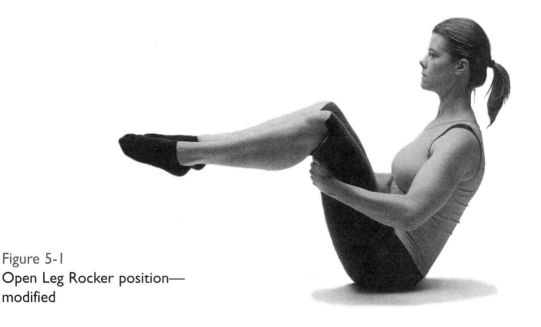

Figure 5-1
**Open Leg Rocker position— modified**

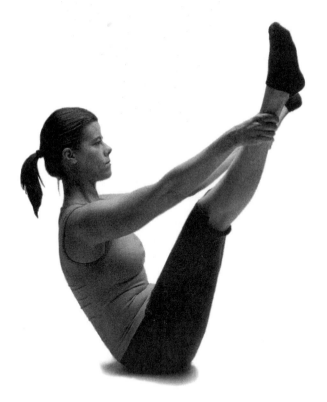

Figure 5-2
Open Leg Rocker position

## NOTES AND GOALS

♦ If this exercise is difficult you can modify it by holding underneath your thighs and keeping your legs bent (see Figure 5-1).

♦ Your lifted chest and "withers" with an elongated lower back, combined with your ribs held in place, will create poise and position on your horse.

♦ Keep a sense of your shoulder blades pressing back and down, not pinching together.

♦ If you are tight, this exercise could be difficult. Modify the exercise by keeping your feet on the floor to find your position. Then extend only one leg to the side, bringing it back down to the floor before extending the second leg.

## SAW (INTERMEDIATE)

This exercise creates flexibility and the ability to rotate the spine while keeping the pelvis (seat) stabilized. It will help you understand how to keep the positioning of your seat bones in the saddle while the twisting of the torso above the waist, which is required for lateral work such as shoulder-in and half pass.

## STEP ONE

Just as you did with the "Spine Stretch Forward" exercise, sit with your legs out in front of you about 3 feet apart. Your ankles should be flexed, but be sure your heels are on the floor. If you are tight, keep your knees bent. Your arms will reach out to the side, however, keep your elbows and hands slightly in front of your shoulders so you can easily see them in your peripheral vision.

## STEP TWO

Inhaling, squeeze your bottom and pull your stomach in and up, feeling your whole spine lengthen from the tailbone stretching down, up through the spine through the "withers" to the back of your neck and out the top of your head. Keeping both seat bones evenly "in the saddle," rotate your torso to the right. As you do this, rotate the right arm inward in the shoulder socket to protect the shoulder joint. Feel that your Box is square as you turn, meaning that your shoulders are level with your hips. This is important later when you use this movement to perform a circle or shoulder-in when mounted.

## STEP THREE

As you exhale, go deep and round beginning with the top of your head reaching for your right knee while the little finger of your left hand reaches toward the little toe of your right foot. Reach your right arm to the opposite diagonal behind

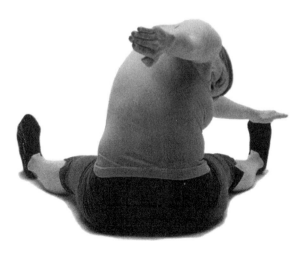

Figure 5-3
Saw

you. This is, in essence, the Spine Stretch Forward with a twist. Feel the left side of your body stretch long toward your right foot by anchoring your left seat bone to the floor. Pull your ribs together with your stomach muscles as you twist and use that action to "wring out" all the air out from your lungs.

## STEP FOUR

Inhale as you return to the starting position. Exhale and relax the muscles slightly. Repeat to the left. Perform five to eight repetitions.

## NOTES AND GOALS

♦ This is another breathing exercise. Utilize your abdominals to press the air out of your lungs, deepening the stretch and the rotation of your spine.

♦ Your little finger may not touch your little toe at first. However, it is more important to keep both seat bones "in the saddle." You will find that as you twist right, your left seat bone will want to lift off the ground. This is an evasion of the stretch! Keep your seat bones firmly planted on the floor.

# SIDE KICKS (INTERMEDIATE)

There are many Side Kick exercises in the Pilates system. To perform them, your Pilates Box is flipped on its side. The force of the movement of the legs, combined with the differing effect of gravity on the Pilates Box on its side, creates a new challenge for the Powerhouse. This exercise will help you understand the concept of independent seat and legs in that it asks you to have a long, swinging, loose leg, but that you keep your pelvis and trunk, i.e., "seat," quiet. The position for all Side Kick exercises is the same.

## THE SIDE KICK POSITION

Lying on your side, align your head, shoulders, ribs and pelvis in a straight line. Feel one shoulder directly over the other shoulder and one hip directly over your other hip. You may hold your head up with your hand, or you may lay your head down on your arm or place a pillow under your head. Move your legs out in front of you in a straight line at approximately a 45-degree angle from your hips. Generate the stance used in Pilates: toes apart and heels together. Keep your knees soft and feet long. Stabilize this position by engaging your Powerhouse and your Box muscles by "feeling your shoulders moving down to meet your stomach in your lower back." Also be sure your back remains wide by keeping your ribs in with your stomach. This stabilization is of the utmost importance because the ensuing exercises will challenge the Box in this side-lying position.

If you are performing all of these, you may complete them all on the first side before turning over to perform the second side.

# FRONT AND BACK

This Pilates exercise is good for those who need more hamstring and hip flexibility. For tight people, try to get as full a range of motion as possible. If you are very flexible, try to make the range of motion very small and concentrate on the Box being perfectly square and stable.

## STEP ONE

Lying in the Side Kick position on your right side, lift your left leg slightly so your foot is level with your hip. Keep your feet in the "heels together, toes apart" position. Wrap your left thigh around like a one-legged wringer washing machine. Be sure your knees remain soft.

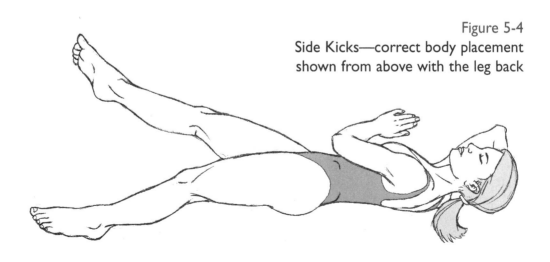

Figure 5-4
Side Kicks—correct body placement
shown from above with the leg back

## STEP TWO

With your Powerhouse engaged, inhale and "swing" your left leg to the front. Maintain your leg position parallel to the floor. Be sure your Box does not sway. Your left shoulder will be inclined to evade the strength and stretch required of this movement by leaning back behind the body as the leg swings forward. Feel your thigh swinging the leg long and loose, as opposed to a tight, stiff leg with a locked knee.

## STEP THREE

Exhale and swing your left leg carefully behind you, activating your left gluteals. Maintain the leg position parallel to the floor. When you actively squeeze your bottom and pull your stomach in and up, you should feel a stretch across your thigh. Be sure your Box does not sway. Your left shoulder will now want to incline forward. Resist this impulse and remain square. You may repeat this 10 times front and back.

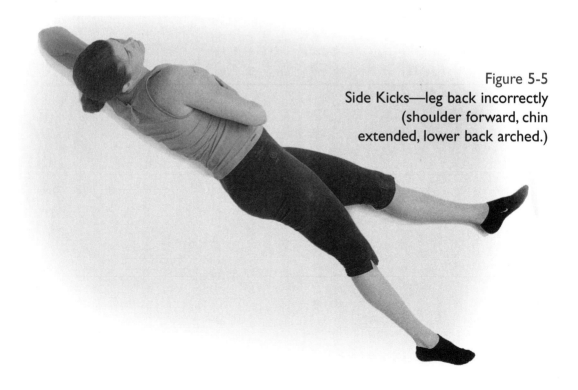

Figure 5-5
Side Kicks—leg back incorrectly
(shoulder forward, chin
extended, lower back arched.)

## NOTES AND GOALS

♦ Be sure to perform this exercise on both sides.

♦ Keeping the Powerhouse engaged while swinging your leg is key. Do not allow your shoulder to rock back and forth to accommodate the movement in your leg (See Figure 5-5).

♦ Later, you may add a pulse of the leg. When the leg reaches the end range of motion, you will relax it for a split second then kick again toward the end range of motion again before swinging back. You may also perform this second pulse when the leg is behind you.

# CIRCLES

This exercise is good for riders with hypermobile knee joints. It strengthens the Box as well as all of the muscles around the hip. Done well, it can help "train" a hypermobile knee to stay soft while the Powerhouse is engaged. There is no breathing pattern to this exercise, but remember to exhale!

## STEP ONE

Lying in the Side Kick position on your right side, lift your left leg slightly so your foot is at the same level as your hip, keeping your knee soft. Think of the left heel turning toward the ground and the toe toward the ceiling.

## STEP TWO

Make a small circle with your left leg by first trying to touch the left heel to the instep of the right foot. From there, circle your leg forward and then up to the starting position, then back down to the instep. The circle should be no larger than a volleyball. Feel as though it is actually your hip circling your thigh rather than your lower leg circling your foot. Make five circles in a forward-moving direction.

## STEP THREE

Reverse the circle, reaching your left leg first down to the instep of the right foot, and then circle your leg backward to start the circles. Repeat five times.

## Notes and goals

♦ Feel your leg circling from the hip and not from the foot or knee.

♦ When you feel you can keep the Powerhouse engaged and the Box stabilized you may try these at a nice brisk tempo.

# Up and Down

This exercise will work the hip and inner and outer thighs. On the way up, the outer thigh requires strength while the inner thigh stretches. On the way down, in addition to the outer thigh working against gravity you also will strengthen the inner thigh by wrapping it with the use of the gluteals and hip adductors. Your knee must remain soft with the movement coming from the hips. Flexing and pointing your feet will work your ankle.

## Step One

Lie in the Side Kick position on your right side. Be sure your heels are together with your toes apart. Maintain soft knees.

## Step Two

Inhaling, lift your left leg up toward the ceiling keeping your knee soft and your foot long. Your knee and toes of the left leg will be pointing toward the ceiling, while the heel will be aimed toward the floor. Be sure that when you lift your leg the integrity of the Box is not compromised.

## Step Three

Exhale as you flex your foot at the ankle. Keeping your knee soft, reach your leg long out of your hips while engaging your bottom. As your leg comes down, feel it pull toward the leg on the ground by wrapping your inner thigh with your gluteals and hip adductors. Feel as though you are trying to move a 1000-pound horse with your inner thigh. Think of reaching the left foot to the instep of the right foot from the hip muscles. Repeat three times.

## Step Four

Keeping your left foot flexed, lift your leg toward the ceiling. With the same instructions as in Step Three, point your left foot as you reach the leg down. Repeat three times.

## NOTES AND GOALS

♦ Be sure to repeat this exercise with the right leg.

♦ As in the preceding exercises, the stability of the Box is more important than the range of motion of your leg. As you lift your leg up, your hip will want to fall back behind you. Resist this evasion by pulling your stomach in and up and using your bottom to press your hips forward.

♦ Keep thinking long in the spine, with length from head to toe. Keep your focus forward to keep your spine aligned.

♦ Tighter people can try to lift their leg higher to increase flexibility in the hips and legs. More flexible or hypermobile people should concentrate on keeping the Box very stable.

♦ Keep your shoulders continually moving back and down toward your lower back.

# INTERMEDIATE MAT EXERCISES LYING ON THE STOMACH

When lying on your stomach, it is very difficult to feel the engagement of your abdominals. Like horses that invert because their abdominals are not engaged, the human back will also hollow and shorten when lying on the stomach if the Powerhouse is not engaged. We can, however, train our abdominals to be engaged even though they may be in a lengthened position. The ability to do this gives us the opportunity to work on strengthening the back muscles, includ-

# HEADS UP!

Keep you Powerhouse engaged! If you feel any discomfort in your lower back with either of the next two exercises, you are not yet strong enough to perform them! Consult your Pilates instructor, doctor or physical therapist for help with these exercises.

ing the mid and lower trapezius, while keeping the lower back safe. In this position, we also can work to lengthen the muscles that flex the hip, allowing for a longer lower back and a more open hip angle.

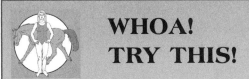

## WHOA! TRY THIS!

Standing, relax all your Powerhouse muscles and lean back from your hips as if you were trying to look up at the ceiling behind you. You will probably feel a pinching in your lower back. Now stay there and soften your knees, squeeze your bottom and pull your stomach in. When engaged, the support of the Powerhouse muscles combined with soft knees will take the pinch out of this movement by keeping your lower back lengthened.

## SINGLE LEG KICK

This exercise opens the chest, elongates the front of the body, and strengthens the back. When done correctly, you will feel a stretch across your thigh and hip flexors. In addition, you will strengthen your mid and lower trapezius, which are important muscles for riding. Using your arms correctly will firm your triceps.

### STEP ONE
Lie on your stomach and lift your upper body onto your elbows. Make a circle with your arms on the floor in front of you as if you were hugging a grocery bag close to you. Making fists, plant the little fingers on the floor and press your forearms into the floor as you lift your chest. Engage your Powerhouse and try to lift your stomach in and up so that it doesn't touch the floor. Pull your shoulders down, meeting your stomach in your lower back. Squeeze your bottom to

elongate your legs with heels together, toes apart. Be sure the front of your hips are on the floor and that you keep your knees soft.

## Step Two

Bend your right knee as if you were going to kick yourself in the bottom. Pulse the bent knee twice. As you do this, your body will evade the stretch across your thigh and hip by releasing the squeeze in your bottom and letting the abdominals go. Be aware of this and keep your Powerhouse engaged.

## Step Three

As you lower your right leg back to the floor, simultaneously bend your left knee and repeat with your left leg. Make sure you don't evade the work of the Powerhouse during the transition! Repeat five to eight times with each leg.

## Step Four

Finish this exercise by curling up into a ball, either on your back, or sit back over your heels and rest your lower back.

## Notes and goals

♦ REMEMBER: If you feel any discomfort in your lower back during this exercise, it is not safe for you to perform it without seeking professional help.

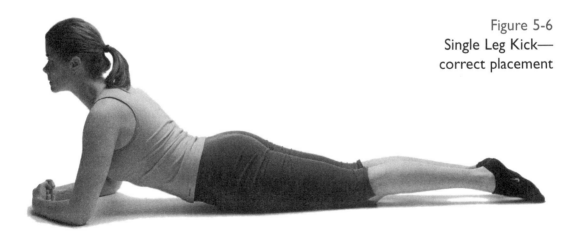

Figure 5-6
Single Leg Kick—
correct placement

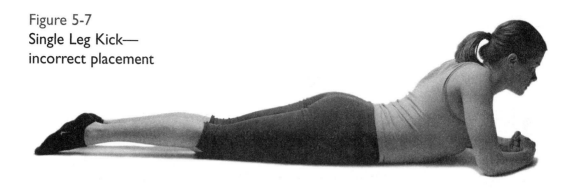

Figure 5-7
Single Leg Kick—
incorrect placement

♦ Be sure your hip bones stay on the floor as you kick one leg. The tendency will be for your hips to rock from side to side. If they do, your Powerhouse is losing engagement.

♦ If you don't feel a stretch across your thigh and the front of your hip, go slowly and be sure your stomach is scooping in and up and your bottom is engaged.

♦ Keep your chest lifted and look straight ahead with an elongated neck. Do not allow your chest to sink, causing your neck to shorten so that the back of your head touches the upper back (See Figure 5-7).

♦ Your breathing will be timed with the leg action. In the beginning you may inhale as you kick one leg and exhale as you kick the other. When you have control over this exercise, you may inhale as you kick both the right and left legs and exhale as you kick each of them again.

# DOUBLE LEG KICK

This exercise is a continuation of the work performed in the Single Leg Kick. You will be required to maintain even more control over your Powerhouse and Box so you can elongate the front of your body without feeling any discomfort in your lower back.

## STEP ONE

Lie on your stomach and place your right cheek on the floor. Clasp your hands behind your back, and bend your elbows to allow your hands to be as high up

# HEADS UP!

This exercise places the shoulder joint in an extreme outward rotated position. If you have any shoulder problem or feel any discomfort in your shoulders when performing this exercise, stop immediately and consult your Pilates instructor, doctor or physical therapist.

on your back as possible. Engage your Powerhouse, but allow your shoulders to be rounded and relaxed. Your elbows will relax toward the ground and your legs will be long with soft knees and your heels together, toes apart.

## STEP TWO
Engage the Powerhouse as you bend both knees to "kick" your bottom three times. As you do so, you will need to pull your abdominals farther in and up to keep your lower back lengthened. Keep your bottom engaged so the front of your hips are pressing into the floor.

## STEP THREE
Return your legs to the floor and, as you do, inhale and slide your clasped hands down your back, reaching your arms toward your feet. Allow your upper back to come off the floor to follow your hands moving toward your feet and look forward. Pull your shoulder blades together and down, and feel your armpits moving toward your waistline. Do not hyperextend your elbows to perform this movement. Rather, feel the reach downward of the arms coming from the shoulder and mid and lower trapezius. Keep your feet on the floor with your knees soft.

## STEP FOUR
Exhale and turn your face to the right and place your left cheek on the floor. Return your hands to their starting position and allow your shoulders to soften and round. As you do so, bend your knees and kick three times. Repeat five to eight times.

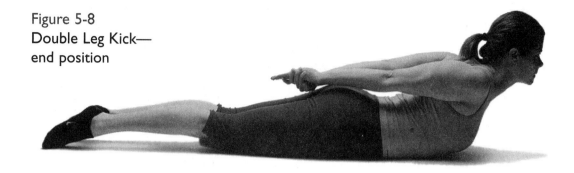

Figure 5-8
Double Leg Kick—
end position

## STEP FIVE

Finish this exercise by curling up into a ball, either on your back, or sit back over your heels and rest your lower back.

## NOTES AND GOALS

♦ REMEMBER: If you feel any discomfort in your shoulders or lower back during this exercise it is not safe for you to perform it without seeking professional help.

♦ When you lift your head and shoulders off the floor, keep your chest and feet on the floor. This will help you keep your Powerhouse engaged so that you use the correct back muscles. Lifting the chest too high off the floor will result in using the lower back instead of the shoulders.

♦ Be sure your shoulder blades not only pinch together, but that they reach down. This will target the mid and lower trapezius.

♦ Keep your knees and elbows soft. When reaching with your arms, it is easy to hyperextend your elbows rather than stretch your arms from your shoulders. Watch for this and, instead, reach back and down with your shoulders.

# SELECTED PILATES EXERCISES FROM THE SYSTEM

The preceding exercises are from intermediate (First and Second Level) mat exercises. Pilates, however, advances past First Level to FEI, if you will. The System requires the practitioner to master the basics and then perform versions of the basics in more complex ways using a variety of specialized apparatus, "magic" circles, arm weights and even a wall. These next exercises, which range from basic to advanced, challenge the basics learned above by asking that the Powerhouse be engaged while standing and sitting.

# THE WALL

The Wall is an exercise that is often used as an end to a full Pilates workout. There are three parts to the Wall. They can follow each other in sequence: Arm Circles, Peeling Off and Skiing. While your mat exercises serve to strengthen, stretch and create symmetry in the body as you lie on the floor, these exercises challenge you to keep symmetry, posture and skeletal alignment while standing. They can help you feel your posture and poise while mounted and help the reader/rider attain an independent seat and hands. Each exercise requires the same stance or posture.

## THE WALL POSTURE

To create the correct Wall posture or stance, your whole spine must be touching the wall, just as the whole spine must touch the floor when you are lying down (See Figure 5-9). To accomplish this, do the following:

## STEP ONE

Stand with your back and feet against a wall, heels together, toes slightly apart. Keep your knees soft and allow your arms to hang loosely at your side. Bring your shoulders back and down, not pinching them together or pressing your arms back. You will notice that your lower back will probably not touch the wall.

## STEP TWO

Engage your Powerhouse. Pull your stomach in and up to press and lengthen your lower spine against the wall. The space between your lower back and the wall should decrease, but probably your back will still not be touching the wall. Engage your bottom so you feel the outward rotation, or the wrapping of your thighs. As you do this, keep your knees soft, even slightly bent if need be. If your back is fully against the wall, you may proceed to the exercise. If not, continue with the following direction.

## STEP THREE

Keeping your Powerhouse engaged, walk your feet away from the wall as needed, up to 8 inches. Your whole spine should now be against the wall. Don't worry if the back of your head is against the wall, but try to keep the chin level. Keep your knees soft.

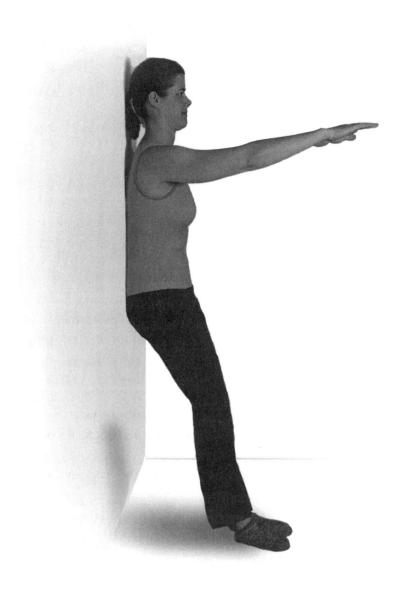

Figure 5-9
The Wall posture

# ARM CIRCLES

Done correctly, you will experience the challenge of moving your arms while your trunk remains quiet and strong. The riding concept of independent seat and hands will become clearer after experiencing this exercise. This exercise works the upper back.

## STEP ONE
Stand in the correct Wall stance. Take a deep breath as you slowly reach your shoulder blades down so your arms can lengthen toward the ground. You will feel here a sense of the armpits moving down to your waistline. This helps you feel the weight of your elbows reaching down that will be useful when riding.

## STEP TWO
Continue to inhale as you reach your energized arms forward out in front of you and continue moving them as high as they can go while the shoulders remain back and down and your whole back remains against the wall. As your arms travel upward, the rib cage and/or lower back will want to come off the wall. Resist this evasion and only take the arms up as high as you can keeping your Powerhouse engaged to keep the whole back against the wall. Be sure your knees remain soft.

## STEP THREE
Exhale as you move your arms to the side and back down to the starting position. Be sure your arms stay in your peripheral vision. Repeat three times and then reverse the pattern.

### NOTES AND GOALS
♦ Keeping the back against wall is the most important part of this exercise.
♦ Be sure to feel your ribs closing inwards as if to push the back of your rib cage into the wall.
♦ Your shoulders must stay down in order to strengthen the mid and lower trapezius.
♦ When reaching your arms to the side, be sure you can see your hands in your peripheral vision. Taking them directly to the side will cause your ribs to pop off the wall and your back to hollow.

♦ As you work this exercise over a period of time, you will want your head to be on the wall. Also work toward getting your feet closer to the wall.

# Peeling Off

The next Wall Exercise is called Peeling Off. This refers to "peeling" the spine off the wall one vertebrae at a time, in effect, performing the mat exercise, the Roll Up, while standing. In order to accomplish this, you must use the Powerhouse to stabilize your lower spine so that it remains against the wall. Not only will this exercise strengthen the Powerhouse, it will supple your spine. You can think of this as another exercise for lengthening and collecting of the spine for the rider!

## Step One

Maintain the Wall stance described above. Beginning with the top of your head, "peel" your spine, one vertebrae at a time off the wall. Do this very slowly with concentration. Begin by bringing your chin to your chest. Your head, like a heavy weight, pulls your neck and shoulders away from the wall. Allow your arms to be relaxed. At this point, double-check your lower back. Be sure it is against the wall by scooping your stomach in and up. Keep your bottom engaged to anchor the stretch of your spine. Feel the wringer washing machine action of your hips and thighs and keep your knees soft. Continue peeling the vertebrae off the wall until you reach your waistline. At this point, it helps to imagine folding your ribs around the lifting in and up of your stomach, to feel the back widen. Breathe with deep inhales and exhales as you go (See Figure 5-10).

## Step Two

Reverse the process and place each vertebrae back on the wall. Maintain the work of the Powerhouse and keep your arms, shoulders and neck relaxed as you use it to place your spine back against the wall. As you place your mid-back against the wall, begin to feel your shoulders gently pulling down into the back. Try to do this without tensing your arms. Repeat 3-4 times.

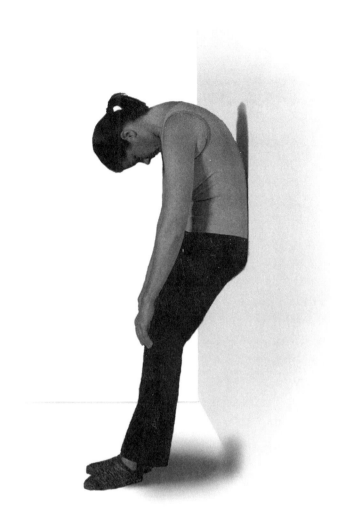

Figure 5-10
Peeling Off

## NOTES AND GOALS

♦ Only go as far as you can maintain your abdominals in and up and your lower back against the wall.

♦ Your shoulders should remain relaxed. Allow gravity to pull them forward and off the wall rather than using muscle effort.

♦ As you place your upper back against the wall, your lower back will try to evade the lengthening by coming off the wall. Be sure you resist this evasion by maintaining the work of your Powerhouse and soft knees.

# SKIING

This exercise should be performed with ease even though it is working on strength. Instead of standing against the wall with your heels together and toes apart, open your feet so they are parallel with each other and move them 10 to 12 inches away from the wall. If needed, your head can be off the wall, but keep your chin level. This exercise will strengthen your bottom muscles, essential for posting.

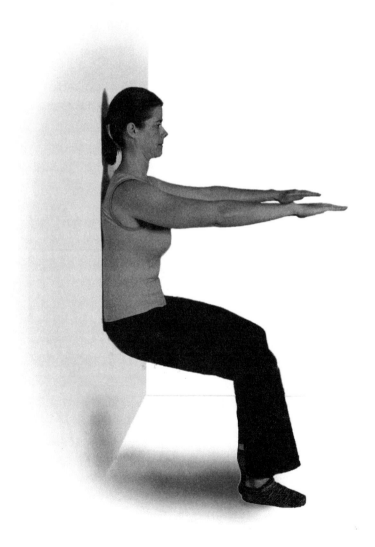

Figure 5-11
Skiing

## STEP ONE

Keeping your whole back against the wall, engage the Powerhouse and slide down the wall until your knees are at right angles with your hips and ankles. As you slide your torso down the wall, keep your shoulders back and down while raising your arms so that they arrive at shoulder level, palms down when the knees reach a right angle. Your knees must aim directly over your toes but not beyond them. Be sure your hips do not go below the level of your knees.

## STEP TWO

Hold this position for a slow five counts while engaging the Powerhouse muscles to be sure the whole back remains against the wall.

## STEP THREE

Deepen the engagement of the Powerhouse (especially your bottom) and straighten your legs from your hips while you press your arms back down to your sides. Be aware that you are using your bottom muscles to straighten the hip to come back up, rather that using your thighs to straighten your knees. See if you can differentiate between these two different ways to straighten your legs. Understanding this difference will help you perceive how to use the Powerhouse to move the body rather than your arms and legs. Repeat this four to six times.

## NOTES AND GOALS

♦ Keeping the back against the wall is the most important part of this exercise.

♦ Be sure to feel your ribs closing inward as if to push the back of your rib cage into the wall.

♦ When you are at the bottom of the "skiing" position, check to be sure your hip, knee and ankle joints make right angles. If they don't, adjust the distance of your feet from the wall accordingly.

♦ Remember to use your haunches to straighten your legs.

# TO FINISH THE WALL EXERCISES

To finish, feel your spine lengthened and flat against the wall by using your Powerhouse. Slowly walk your feet back to the wall, and engage your Powerhouse even more to keep your spine against the wall as your feet come in. When your feet are underneath you, use your arms to help push you away from the wall, and step forward feeling tall.

# CHAIR EXERCISES (FROM THE PILATES "TV EXERCISES")

The sitting Leg Lifts will help the rider weight both seat bones equally in the saddle. Done with attention to precision, it will strengthen the symmetry in the Box by use of the asymmetry in the legs.

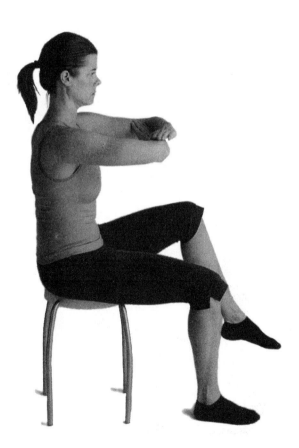

Figure 5-12
Chair exercise—
correct

# LEG LIFTS

Sit in a chair with your feet flat on the floor. Feel your Box balanced over your two seat bones with your stomach working in and up to pull your ribs back, as if they were pressing against a wall. Engage your bottom and feel your shoulders moving back and down to meet your stomach in your lower back. Cross your arms at chest level or rest your arms by your side. If needed, you can hold on to the chair for support. Be sure your shoulders are directly over your hips.

## STEP ONE

Without disturbing your posture, carefully lift your right knee up toward your chest. The knee will, for now, remain bent. Hold for up to a count of five—but only as long as you can hold your body correctly. While holding, revisit your posture to be sure that your Powerhouse is engaged and that both seat bones

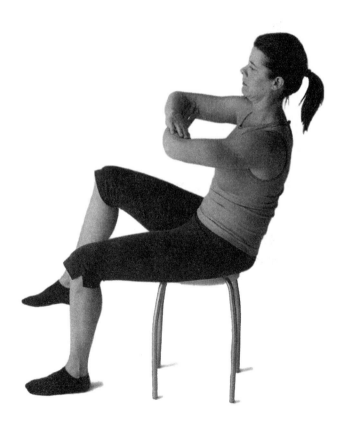

Figure 5-13
Chair exercise—
incorrect

are still square in the "saddle." You should feel your back flat as if against a wall, while the sides of your body remain lifted and lengthened.

## Step Two

If you are able to maintain the balanced posture, instead of holding your knee bent, slowly extend your lower leg from the knee. Be sure your shoulders are not leaning back behind your hips or off to one side when you attempt this. As you extend your lower leg, feel your stomach moving even farther back to keep your whole back long as if it were against a wall.

## Step Three

Bend your knee and place your right leg back on the floor. Repeat with your left leg. Perform this exercise five times on each leg.

## Notes and goals

♦ When you lift your right leg, you will be tempted to shift your weight to your left seat bone. Resist this and remain square.

♦ Your back must remain as if it were against a wall. When your leg is lifted, you will be tempted to counterbalance the weight of the leg by leaning backward (See Figure 5-13). If this happens, keep your knee bent until you can build the strength to hold the Box straight and strong while you extend the leg.

# Exercises from the Pilates Standing Arm Weight Series

Both of the following exercises require a similar stance to that used in the Wall exercise. The difference is that now you are not standing against a wall. To help keep the feeling of having your back against the wall, incline your shoulder girdle slightly in front of your hips with your arms hanging loosely at your sides. Shift your weight slightly forward onto the balls of your feet. Engage your Powerhouse to energize and lengthen your spine, and feel as though you are pressing your whole back against a wall. Anchor this posture with your bottom to encourage your lower back to lengthen. Keep your knees soft and your bottom tight so that your upper thighs are wrapping around like an old-fashioned wringer washing machine. These exercises are normally performed with a one pound weight in each hand, however they are described here without using weights. If you choose to use weights, be sure they are only one pound, since the idea of the Pilates Arm Weight series is to create resistance within the muscles as opposed to just lifting a weight.

# SIDE BEND (INTERMEDIATE)

This exercise is not unlike what you ask your horse to do when asking for him to bend his whole body. You will experience the importance of keeping the Powerhouse engaged while bending in order to control the whole spine and experience the full benefit of the exercise. Exercising with precision is a must in order to perform the Side Bend of the spine safely. To do this, it is important to keep your shoulder girdle slightly in front of your hips with your Powerhouse engaged. Also be sure that your rib cage does not collapse down onto the hip (popping the shoulder out) but, rather, feel it lift up and over to the side.

## STEP ONE
Stand as described above. Without disturbing your Box, lift your right arm to the ceiling as you inhale. The shoulder is allowed to rise up slightly so that your elbow is close to the head. If your Powerhouse is engaged, you will feel a lengthening in your side from your waistline to shoulder.

## STEP TWO
Exhale as you reach your right arm to the left and bend your spine to the left while keeping your shoulders inclined slightly in front of your hips. Imagine that you are laying your spine sideways up and over a beach ball. You will be inclined to evade the stretch by moving your hips or ribs to the right and collapsing the left side of your body. Watch for this "popping out" of the hips and ribs, and anchor the movement by keeping the lower back lengthened with your Powerhouse with your knees soft. You will feel how much evasion of the stretch can make this exercise seem easier than it really is. Revisit your stomach and be sure it is in and up, pushing your rib cage back so your back doesn't hollow.

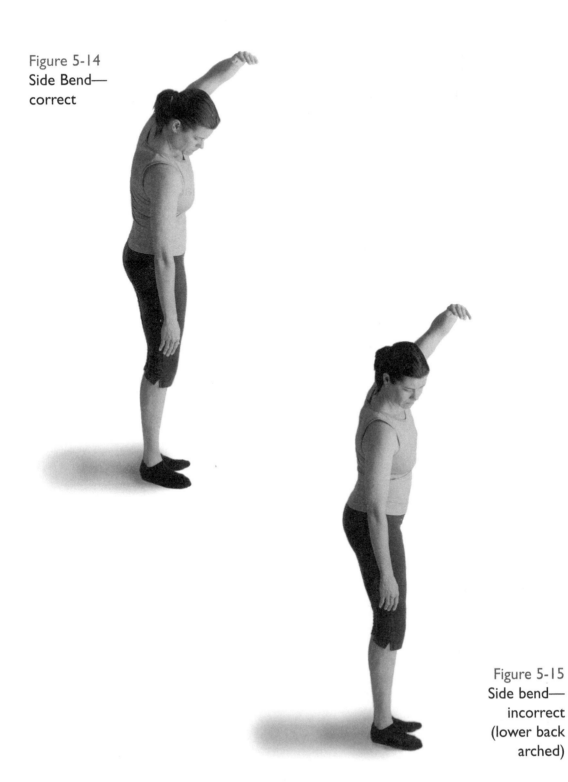

Figure 5-14
Side Bend—
correct

Figure 5-15
Side bend—
incorrect
(lower back
arched)

## STEP THREE

To come back to straight, inhale and deepen the engagement of your Powerhouse as you restack the vertebrae, one by one, from the side bend to an upright position with your head being the last part up. Exhale and relax. Repeat on the other side. Perform this up to five times on each side.

## NOTES AND GOALS

♦ You will experience more stretch with your stomach muscles maximally engaged.

♦ When you reach your arm to the side, keep a sense of reaching from the back of your armpit through your elbow and out the hand. This will allow both sides of the body to elongate even more. Your elbow will want to bend to avoid the lengthening of the sides of the back. Keep it straight but be sure the joint is not locked.

♦ Do not arch your lower back. It is essential that you keep your shoulder girdle just in front of your hips. This slight lean forward, combined with the engagement of your Powerhouse to anchor the pelvis, will not only keep your lower back safe, but also serve to deepen the stretch (See Figure 5-15).

# CHEST EXPANSION (ADVANCED)

This exercise is essential for the rider. It exemplifies the work in the mid and lower trapezius while stabilizing the core, which is necessary for the basic dressage position. In Chapter 7, it will be called on to help the rider understand how to use her core to assist in many dressage movements.

The movement in this exercise is seemingly simple, but it will challenge the Powerhouse to keep the Box intact. If the exercise seems easy, you can be assured that your Powerhouse is probably not completely engaged and that there is some evasion.

## STEP ONE

Stand as described for the Side Bend exercise but reach your arms directly in front of your shoulders at shoulder height. Engage your Powerhouse and pull your shoulders down into your back, feeling them meet your stomach in your lower back. Shift your weight slightly onto the balls of your feet with your bottom anchoring the tailbone down so the lower back can lengthen.

## Step Two

As you inhale to expand your chest, draw your arms straight down past your sides and reach behind your hips. Feel your shoulder blades pulling together and down to open your chest. Your hands should feel as though they are pressing back against a wall. The evasion of this exercise occurs when the ribs pop out to the front or the shoulders round in. Resist these and keep your ribs pressing back with your stomach in and up while your shoulders pull back and down to open your chest. Keep your bottom tight, your upper thighs "wrapping" and your knees soft.

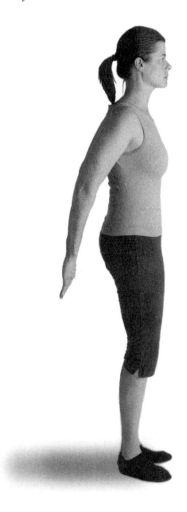

Figure 5-16
Chest Expansion

## STEP THREE

As you are holding your breath, turn your head to look over your right shoulder, then turn and look over your left shoulder, then return your focus straight ahead. Your neck should remain relaxed so that your head can turn from side to side without tension. Keep the Powerhouse deeply engaged, and keep the knees soft.

## STEP FOUR

Exhale as you return your arms to the starting position. As you do this feel your fingertips reach farther down to the floor. This will encourage the mid and lower trapezius to work to keep your shoulders back and down. It will also give you a sense of your armpits moving down toward your waistline—the feeling necessary for keeping your elbows anchored while riding. Repeat four times, alternating the look to the opposite shoulder.

## NOTES AND GOALS

♦ Moving your arms back behind your shoulders will cause your ribs to move forward, allowing your mid and low back to hollow. Your shoulders will want to round forward, the exact opposite of the desired end goal of the exercise. Both of these are evasions of the exercise that must be resisted.

♦ Your back must remain as if it were against a wall. As your arms move back, your stomach needs to work harder to keep your ribs from popping forward.

♦ Remember, if this exercise seems easy, you have probably allowed the body to evade the exercise in some way.

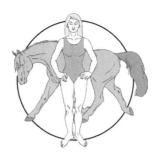

# CHAPTER 6
# MOUNTED PILATES EXERCISES

Although Joseph Pilates was not a rider, nor did he create exercises specifically for riders, the Pilates exercises done while mounted are developed from the exercises in preceding chapters. I have readjusted these mat and selected exercises from the Pilates System so they can be executed while on top of a horse. In doing so, I hope to provide the rider with not only a warm-up for her body before setting to work, but also a basis for using the musculature learned through the preceding Pilates exercises while mounted for later riding explorations.

As stated above, each exercise is one that you have already learned in Chapters 4 and 5 that is now adapted to a sitting position on the horse. It is my intention that you have correctly mastered the basic and advancing Pilates exercises at home first. Then, before trying these mounted, you will have practiced them at home in a chair. As you walk around the arena to let your horse loosen up before going to work, you can use that time to work on your body.

These mounted exercises should be performed in an enclosed area. You will need a trustworthy mount, calm enough to walk on a loose rein and not be disturbed by movement in the saddle. If there is any question about control over the horse, have someone experienced lunge you while you perform the exercises, first at a walk. When they become easy and your horse is not disturbed, they may be tried on the lunge at the trot.

# Starting Position

Your position in the saddle must remain the same for all exercises. Unless otherwise directed to do so, place both hands on the pommel to help stabilize your torso, with the reins loosely in your hands. Allow your legs to hang loosely at the sides of your horse with your feet in or out of the stirrups. As with the Chair Exercise in Chapter 5, you will want to sit up straight with your Powerhouse lightly engaged. Your shoulders will be directly over your hips so you can feel your Box square and balanced over your two seat bones. Feel your shoulders pulling back and down to meet your stomach in your lower back. Engage your bottom and feel the slight scoop of your pelvis and a gentle wrapping feel of your upper thighs. Your Powerhouse should feel tight and solid, but not tense.

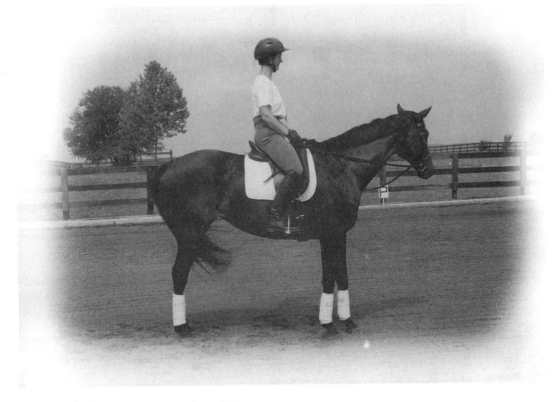

Figure 6-1 Correct mounted position

If you do these exercises at a walk, be sure to use your bottom only enough to help you remain on the saddle symmetrically. You will notice that you will need to use and let go of your Powerhouse dynamically to keep you square in the saddle. This is the essence of being strong and not stiff. You will use muscle tension only to support your position as needed. Too much will create stiffness and loss of balance. Too little use of your Powerhouse and you will be at the mercy of every step the horse takes.

If you are not sure you are square, use a mirror or friend to help you feel the position.

# HUNDREDS

Like the Hundreds in Chapter 4, this exercise will help get the breath flowing through your body. If you keep your Powerhouse muscles engaged, your spine will begin to stretch and lengthen.

## STEP ONE
Sit on your horse as described in the Starting Position with your horse standing still or walking. Breathe in deeply for five counts and exhale for five counts. Keep your abdominals in while you inhale and pull them in farther while you exhale. During the exercise remember to feel your sitting position as described above. Perform 10 breaths.

# SPINE STRETCH FORWARD/WALL PEELING OFF

Refer back to either the Spine Stretch Forward in Chapter 4 or the Wall Peeling Off in Chapter 5. Performing either one will help the reader/rider learn to articulate the spine in a stretch forward. This is a "deep and round" exercise for the rider.

## STEP ONE
Sit on your horse as described in the Starting Position. Take a deep breath in.

## STEP TWO

As you exhale, peel the spine forward, as if coming off a wall. Lower your chin to your chest allowing the crown of your head to lead your spine toward the pommel of the saddle. Feel your ribs fold in, your shoulders relax and your abdominals pull toward your lower back. This is the rider's feeling of working "deep and round." Think of making a C-curve of the spine. Keep your bottom engaged to anchor your seat in the saddle, which will aid to stretch out your lower back and keep the seat bones pointing slightly forward.

## STEP THREE

Inhale and unfold your spine, using your abdominals to "stack" the vertebrae on top of each other one at a time, with a feeling of pressing your spine back on to the wall. Use your Powerhouse to keep your spine engaged as it lengthens back to straight. Exhale and relax. Repeat five times.

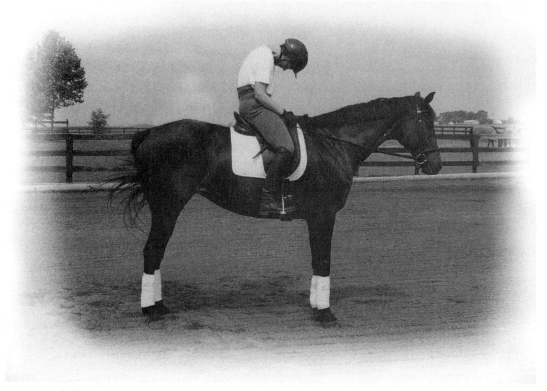

Figure 6-2 **Spine Stretch Forward**

# ARM CIRCLES (FROM THE WALL EXERCISES)

Unless you have a very safe and trustworthy mount, this exercise is best done on the lunge line since you will not be able to use your reins. By maintaining the sitting position as described and allowing your arms to move with ease, you will be able to understand how your hands and arms can be independent from your seat that is being stabilized with your Powerhouse/Box muscles. If it is not possible to perform this exercise with both arms simultaneously, you may modify this exercise by using one arm at a time.

## STEP ONE
Sit on your horse as described in the Starting Position. Let your reins hang loose or knot them for this exercise, and allow your arms to hang loosely by your sides.

## STEP TWO
Inhale as you reach your fingertips down toward the ground, feeling your hands pulling your shoulder blades back and down. With your shoulders continually pulling down, reach your arms forward toward your horse's ears. Since you are not standing against a wall, it will be difficult to tell if you have allowed your rib cage to move forward as your arms move forward and up. Therefore, as your arms move forward, concentrate on keeping your rib cage actively moving back by keeping your stomach moving in and up as though you were standing against the wall.

## STEP THREE
When you have reached your arms as high as they can go with your shoulders down and ribs back, exhale and reach your arms toward the side and back down to the ground. Keep your hands in your peripheral vision as they reach to the side. Check your stomach and be sure it is lifting in and up and that your lower back remains long by using your bottom muscles. Return your arms to a relaxed position hanging loosely at your sides.

## STEP FOUR
Repeat three times and reverse the arm pattern. Your ability to do this exercise correctly—meaning moving your arms without disturbing your back—will help keep your seat and back strong while you use your rein aids.

# LEG LIFTS (FROM THE PILATES CHAIR EXERCISES)

The Leg Lift is exactly the same exercise as the Leg Lifts in Chapter 5. Try this exercise at the halt first. If you are secure, you may try it at the walk. This exercise will help you feel your seat bones evenly in the saddle.

## STEP ONE

Sit on your horse as described in the Starting Position. Inhale as you carefully lift your right knee toward your chest without disturbing your posture. Pay special attention to the feeling of having both seat bones in the saddle.

## STEP TWO

Exhale and hold the leg for up to a count of five—but only as long as you can hold your body correctly. While holding, revisit your posture. Be sure your stom-

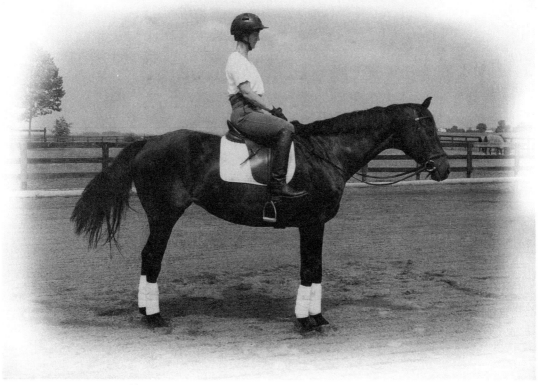

Figure 6-3 **Leg Lifts correct**

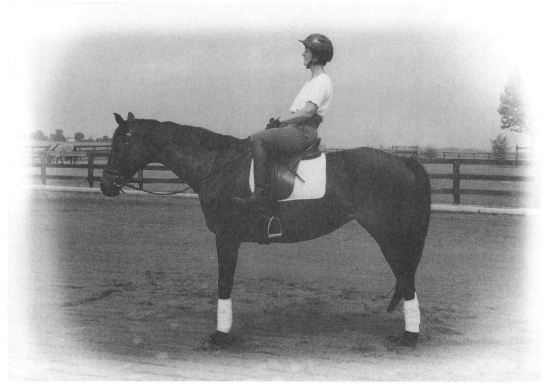

Figure 6-4 Leg Lifts incorrect

ach is lifting in and up and your bottom is lightly engaged. It is important to be sure that your shoulders are not tilting back or listing to one side. When you lift your right leg, you will be tempted to shift your weight to your left seat bone. Resist this and remain square. Also be sure not to lean back to counter balance the weight of your leg.

## STEP THREE

Inhale as you lower your leg and exhale as you revisit your posture. Repeat with the left leg. Repeat four times each leg.

# SIDE BEND (FROM THE PILATES ARM WEIGHT SERIES)

You performed this exercise in Chapter 5 (Figure 5-14) while standing. This exercise will lengthen the sides of the back.

## STEP ONE

Sit on your horse as described in the Starting Position. Incline your shoulder girdle slightly in front of your hips while keeping your rib cage actively moving back. You can feel this if you think of closing your ribs in toward each other. Place both reins in your left hand and place your left hand on the pommel.

## STEP TWO

Inhale as you lift your right arm up to the sky. Allow your shoulder to gently come up so you can feel the reach of the arm coming from your waistline.

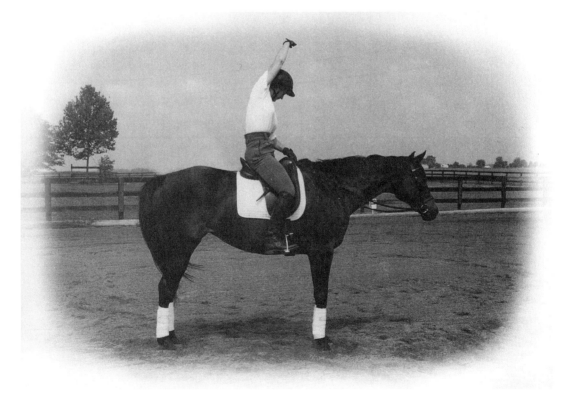

Figure 6-5 **Side Bend**

## STEP THREE

Exhale as you bend to the left, reaching your right arm diagonally forward with your shoulders slightly in front of your hips. Feel the rib cage close together so the middle of your back widens. Imagine that you are laying your spine sideways up and over a beach ball. Keep your right seat bone firmly in the saddle. Revisit your Powerhouse and lift your stomach in and up again. You will experience more stretch by anchoring your seat in the saddle with the engagement of the bottom and your abdominals maximally engaged.

## STEP FOUR

To come back to straight, inhale as you anchor the right seat bone again. Pull your stomach in and up and restack the vertebrae one by one to an upright position. Your head will be the last part up. Exhale when you are upright and lower the right arm to the pommel. Repeat to the other side. Repeat three times to each side.

## VARIATION

If your mount can be trusted, perform the same exercise with the arm that was on the pommel, instead, hanging loosely at your side. At the end of the bend to the left, feel your left arm weighted, as if you had a 3-pound weight in your hand. Repeat on the other side with the same image.

# TWISTING (THIS IS THE FIRST PART OF THE SAW)

Mastering this exercise is essential for circles and all lateral work such as shoulder-in and half pass. It educates the body to firmly stabilize the seat in the saddle as you rotate your trunk above the waist to match your shoulders with the horse's.

## STEP ONE

Sit on your horse as described in the Starting Position. Feel both seat bones firmly in the saddle. Place your reins in your left hand at the pommel. Take a deep breath in as you lift your stomach in and up and turn your rib cage and shoulders to the right. As you turn, be sure your left seat bone remains firmly in the saddle and your sternum lifts so that your shoulders can remain even, i.e., that the rib cage does not collapse on one side and lift on the other. Feel your shoulders pressing down to meet your stomach in your lower back.

## STEP TWO

Staying in the twist, exhale while pulling your stomach back more toward your spine as you are twisting your torso farther to the right as if you were trying to look behind you moving your right hand to the cantle. Continue to engage your bottom to lengthen your lower back and keep your seat bones firmly in the saddle. Feel your shoulders blades continually moving back and down. Holding on to the saddle at the pommel and cantle can help you feel the anchoring of your seat bones into the saddle and encourage you to stay square as you twist even more.

## STEP THREE

Inhale as you slowly return to center. Exhale and revisit your posture. Repeat to the other side. This can be done three times to each side.

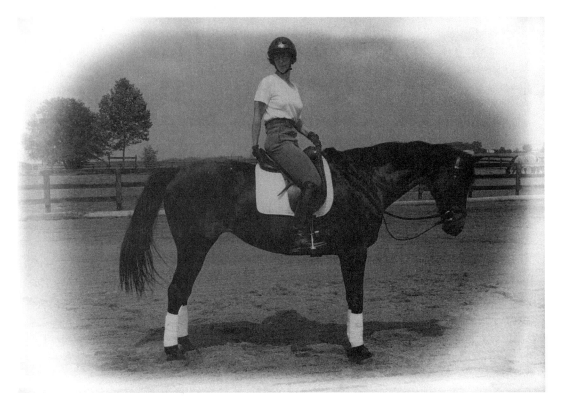

Figure 6-6 Twisting

# ARCHING

This exercise is essentially the positioning of the upper back that you performed in Single Leg Kick and Double Leg Kick in Chapter 5 Figures 5-6 and 5-8. Although this exercise has no direct use in dressage, it does work your shoulder blades back and down to open your chest, which will help you to feel your spine lengthened without shortening your back. It will inform your Basic Dressage Position and will be of use when experimenting with lengthenings, both of which are explained in Chapter 7.

## STEP ONE

Sit on your horse as described in the Starting Position. Take a deep breath in. As you exhale, slowly lift your face and sternum toward the sky. Your ribs will want to go forward, your back will want to hollow and your seat bones will want to tip toward the horse's tail. Resist this evasion. Instead, feel your lower back elongate by scooping your stomach in and up while your bottom engages to deepen your tailbone into the saddle. This dynamic stabilization of the Powerhouse will keep your seat bones anchored, tipping slightly forward toward the horse's head. Press your shoulder blades down to meet your stomach in your lower back, and pull your ribs in toward each other.

## HEADS UP!

Take the same cautions in this exercise as in the exercises that are performed lying on your stomach. You must be able to perform this exercise with NO discomfort in your lower back. If you feel any discomfort in your lower back, you must stop. This means that you are not strong enough to execute the exercise properly. Doing this exercise incorrectly will actually shorten and weaken your back.

## STEP TWO

Inhale and return your face and sternum back to the starting position. Repeat five times.

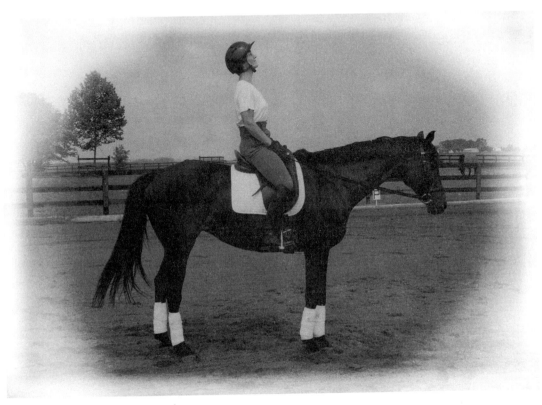

Figure 6-7 **Arching correctly**

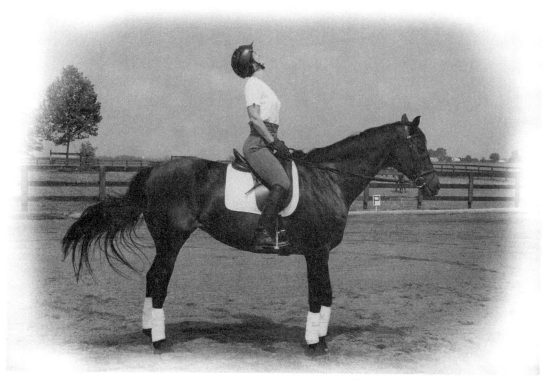

Figure 6-8 Arching incorrectly

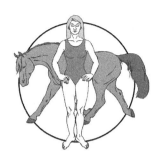

# CHAPTER 7
# PILATES AND DRESSAGE: RIDER EXPLORATION

Mastering an art form is a long process. Dance, martial arts, playing music and dressage all require years of study. Of course, there are the gifted students who seem to be able to quite naturally, perform movements that require physical skill. But for most people, a high level of skill can be attained through good instruction and intense personal study. There are excellent teachers in every discipline, however, very often students are told what to do, and it is up to them to figure out how to do it in the course of their personal explorations. This chapter seeks to help the rider in this arena of study.

In dressage, the utilization of the body knowledge gained through Pilates can help unravel the mystery of how to accomplish the directives of dressage. Here, the thoughts and experiments using Pilates to help achieve particular dressage movements are just that. Your riding instructor is the professional who is teaching you how to ride your horse. However, if the horse and rider have achieved some degree of skill in dressage, it is feasible to assume that the rider can utilize physical abilities gained through the Pilates exercises to help better her riding. This is done by encouraging the reader/rider to explore how to use a learned Pilates exercise to impart clearer aids to her horse. With correct use of muscular tension in specific parts of the Powerhouse and Box, as performed in the preceding Pilates exercises, the rider should eventually be able to use her body more effectively to create balance and harmony between herself and her horse.

The following experiments and thoughts are a guide to help the reader/rider put the Pilates body knowledge to work. The experiments are just a starting point for the reader. It is hoped that the reader will continue further exploration and that through exploration, she will speed her progress toward her dressage goals.

Before you begin your explorations, be sure to take the following under advisement:

♦ You must have gained a solid understanding of the Pilates exercises in the preceding chapters in order to make these explorations viable. Not completely understanding the information in Chapters 2 and 3 will make it difficult to relate the specific exercises or concepts to the exercises being asked of the horse.

♦ Think about the engagement of your muscles as an effort from 1 to 10. One is the lightest muscle contraction, and 10 is the maximum. Experiment with differing amounts of muscle tension, always trying to use the Pilates concept of using the minimum of effort to produce the maximum result. Remember it is the understanding of how to use strength while remaining supple that is key to graceful and seemingly effortless riding.

♦ You will want to try these experiments at home in a chair before attempting to try them mounted. That way you can practice the coordination of isolating the specific muscles for movements without worrying about what your horse is doing.

♦ Understand that the core/trunk muscles can and will be used independently of each other. Most Pilates exercises are performed symmetrically, requiring that all Powerhouse and Box muscles be engaged at the same time to build strength. However, while performing movements required by dressage riding, it is essential that there is a dynamic interplay of these muscles with varying degrees of muscle effort.

♦ Although the head and eyes are not discussed in these experiments, it is expected that the rider look forward keeping the chin level, allowing the head and eyes to direct where the movement is going. The lower leg, also not discussed, should remain long and loose at the horse's side. The hands are equally ignored, and the author assumes the rider will use proper dressage principles to hold and use the reins to communicate softly with the horse's mouth. What is intended is that the reader/rider begin to use her

Pilates knowledge to develop and understand how to find and use a more stabilized and effective seat.

# UNDERSTANDING THE BASIC DRESSAGE POSITION

The proper position for riding dressage is fairly well agreed on. While sitting in the saddle, a plumb line should run from the rider's ear straight down through the middle of her shoulder, rib cage, hip and heel. It is the same proper posture as seen when standing in Chapter 2 Figure 2-2. The only difference in posture is that because the rider is sitting, the knee is bent slightly forward. See Figure 6-1. Unless you have perfect posture, attaining this position while mounted will take muscular effort of the core/trunk muscles. The effort will vary from rider to rider depending on each person's particular skeletal deviations.

## EXPERIMENT WITH THE BASIC DRESSAGE POSITION

A simple, but not easy, way to find how to achieve this basic dressage position is to refer back to the Open Leg Rocker exercise found in Chapter 5 (Figure 5- 2). If you refer to Figure 7-1, you will see a conceptual version of the Open Leg Rocker position performed on top of a horse. This illustration is only to help the reader to visualize the feeling of this exercise while mounted. Of course, when you are mounted, you will have your legs down at the side of your horse. However, the work of the Pilates Box and core muscles should feel exactly as they do when performing the Open Leg Rocker position. The balance necessary to perform this exercise will aid the rider in finding her balance while mounted.

To begin to relate this exercise to the basic dressage position, feel both seat bones firmly in the saddle, weighting each of them equally. Your stomach will be in and up while your bottom gently engages, allowing your spine to elongate from your tailbone up to your withers. Feel how the engagement of the Powerhouse creates a scoop in your pelvis so you are not perched on your seat bones but, rather, you are slightly pointing them toward the horse's withers. It should almost feel like you are trying to sit on your back pockets while also trying to stretch your spine upward. Using your Powerhouse in this way will help you sit deeper in the saddle as opposed to pinching your bottom up and out of the saddle. This scooped position must be maintained by your Powerhouse muscles and will prevent you from tensing and shortening your back.

Next, while maintaining your Powerhouse muscles, engage your main Box muscles—the mid and lower trapezius. To do this, press your shoulders back and down, feeling them meeting your stomach in your lower back. Think back to the Arching exercise in Chapter 6. Although you won't be turning your face upwards, remember the feeling of the sternum lifting while the shoulders are moving back and down. Be careful you don't allow your ribs

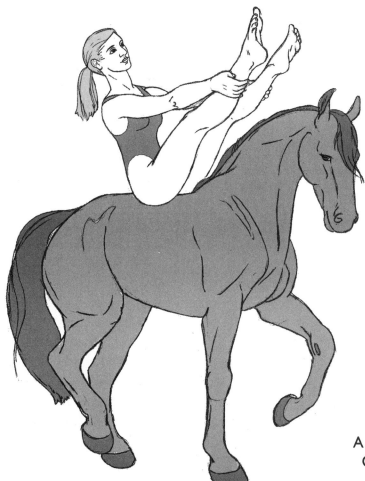

Figure 7-1
A conceptual version of the
Open Leg Rocker Position
while mounted

to poke forward. Rather, counteract that evasion by feeling your mid-back move backward as if you were standing against a wall. If you refer to the Arm Circles in the Wall Exercises in Chapter 5, you will feel your elbows lowering toward the ground with the feeling of your armpits moving down to your waistline. From these downward elbows, allow the energy to flow forward into your hands toward the horse's mouth. Feel the chest open and look straight ahead.

Achieving this position takes a tremendous amount of concentrated effort. Be sure that you are not tensing your muscles and holding your breath. As your posture changes over time using the Pilates exercises, you will find that it takes much less effort to maintain this position.

To find your optimum basic riding position on the horse, as you have probably discovered, is not easy. Add in the fact that once the horse moves, the dynamics of the horse's back creates force on the rider's pelvis. This movement inevitably affects the spine, hence the rider's position. It becomes clear, then, that any instability in the spine or postural deviations from optimum will be accentuated when the horse begins to move. The rider needs to utilize a dynamic muscular effort in order to maintain the proper dressage position when the horse moves. To stabilize the body when the horse is moving, it is essential to think about upward transition, since even moving from a halt to a walk must be considered just that.

## Upward Transitions

It is commonly agreed that, when riding a horse, leg pressure means "go". Unfortunately this usually means that the rider must take her legs off the horse to kick him forward. When the horse does go forward, the rider, who has now probably lost the stability of her position because of this leg movement, will tend to either fall forward or be left behind the horse's center when the horse moves off. Ideally, the horse will move forward from the rider's seat and upper thighs. If this can be accomplished, the lower legs can now lightly hug the horse's sides to maintain a straight and forward direction. To accomplish this, try the following experiment:

## EXPERIMENT WITH UPWARD TRANSITIONS

By experimenting with the engagement of your Powerhouse muscles, you can create a less obvious aid to create the "go" in an upward transition. To ask your horse to move off, first feel your core/trunk muscles active and lightly engaged so that you begin with the stabilized seat of the Open Leg Rocker Position. Then engage your Powerhouse muscles even more to create a deep scoop of the stomach and bottom so that your seat bones and upper thighs send the energy forward. Think back to the wringer-washing machine effect of the thighs explained in Chapter 2, Figure 2-7. Feel how the wrapping around of the thighs inherent in the use of the Powerhouse muscles can contribute to the sense of forward movement of the seat.

At first, you may need to use your lower legs in combination with this seat action. As your horse begins to understand the use of your seat, he may respond by moving forward from this seat action alone. Eventually, this scooping movement of the seat and outward rotation of the upper thigh can serve to replace kicking of the legs to ask the horse to move forward.

When the horse responds, be sure to relax the muscle tension that you used to ask the horse to move forward, but keep enough activation to create a driving seat necessary for the amount of forward for which you asked. With your seat stabilized by control over your core/trunk muscles, your lower legs can remain in light contact with the horse's sides, ready to be used for a more specific aid. Try this to move into a walk and a trot.

## UPWARD CANTER TRANSITION

To achieve the right lead canter we are often instructed to "slide the right seat bone forward." How one accomplishes this can vary. Using the Powerhouse Scoop asymmetrically can help the rider accomplish this with relative simplicity. To ask for the right lead canter, start by using the same directions for moving upward to a walk or trot. However, you will squeeze and scoop your right bottom muscle more. The action of the right gluteus will create a wrapping of the right upper thigh, which will send the right seat bone forward. This isolation of the right bottom can only be effective if the rest of the body, or Box, does not move. To stabilize the Box, actively pull your stomach in and up to keep your spine lengthened and lifted so the horse can more clearly feel the seat bone as it slides forward. Simultaneously, you will need to stabilize your right shoulder back and down with more effort than your left in order to emphasize the specificity of the right seat bone movement. Reverse these actions for the left lead canter.

# PITCHING FORWARD AND FALLING BACK

In upward transitions, the difficulty for the rider is to maintain her center over the horse's. Sometimes the horse will surge forward, leaving the rider behind the motion. Other times the rider will anticipate the upward transition and lean forward thinking she will be with the horse's movement. Another problem occurs when the horse pulls on the reins causing the rider to be unseated. These problems can be addressed by first understanding what actually happens in each situation.

## PITCHING FORWARD/ HORSE PULLING

When the rider pitches forward during an upward transition or when the horse tries to pull the rider out of the saddle, it is usually because the muscles that extend the rider's hip, (gluteus maximus) and the muscles that keep the shoulder girdle anchored to the waistline (mid and lower trapezius) become disengaged. When the bottom muscles release, the hip joint flexes (the angle of the hip decreases), allowing the seat bones to reverse their position from pointing forward toward the withers to pointing backward toward the horse's tail. This tips the waistline forward causing the rider's back and neck to shorten. At the same time, the shoulders are no longer anchored back and down, allowing the rider's shoulder girdle to fall forward toward the horse's neck.

### *THOUGHTS ON PITCHING FORWARD OR BEING PULLED OUT OF THE SADDLE*

You can try to counteract this problem by engaging your Powerhouse and Box muscles more. When you ask your horse to move forward, increase the scoop with your bottom. This will help you maintain an open hip angle and keep your seat bones firmly in place. At the same time use increased muscle effort of the Box muscles to maintain an open chest with your shoulders back and down. Refer back to Chapter 5 and the Arm Circles from the Wall

Exercise. Thinking of pressing your back into a wall while pulling your armpits down into your waistline can help you avoid being pulled forward.

## FALLING BACK

When the rider is left behind during an upward transition, it is usually because the rider's Powerhouse is not engaged. When the horse moves forward, the rider's hip angle is allowed to increase, and the front of the body is elongated. The rider's ribs splay forward as her head and neck fall back behind the hips. Because the rider is behind the movement, the forward movement of the horse's head will pull the rider's arms forward, losing control of keeping the shoulders back and down, which the rider usually tries to counteract by shortening her back even more.

### *THOUGHTS ON FALLING BACK*

To counteract this problem, feel your stomach engaging from the pelvis to the top of your rib cage as if you were wearing a corset. Along with this, feel your spine lengthen even more up through your withers (the back of your neck) to help keep your chin level so the weight of your head does not pull you back. You will need to maintain an open chest by using the increased muscle effort of your shoulders pulling back and down so your elbows keep reaching down to your waistline.

## MAINTAINING BASIC POSITION IN WALK, TROT AND CANTER

Now that the horse is moving forward, the Powerhouse muscles will need to dynamically engage more or less depending on what the motion of the horse does to the rider's body. This is, in essence, dynamically maintaining the Basic Dressage Position. As you walk, trot or canter, notice how much or how little it takes to maintain this position in order feel your seat flowing with the horse without stiffening or collapsing your spine. Maintaining stability during the upward transition as well as in keeping the horse moving forward in any gait will take practice to gain the skill needed to make instant adjustments in the effort of these muscles should you fall behind or get ahead of your horse's movement. If you hold any of these muscles with too much tension, you will create stiffness. If you don't use them enough, you will be left behind or fall forward. The ability of the rider to stabilize her own body will make it possible for the horse to achieve better balance.

# Downward Transitions, Half Halt and Rein-Back

We are often instructed to half halt or halt with our body. Not really knowing what this means, the rider will often lean back and pull on the reins. While this usually serves the purpose, if the rider instead, halts or slows her horse by learning how to use her seat and back with less rein, the movement into the halt becomes more effective and graceful. By exploring the use of the Powerhouse, the rider might find this next experiment helpful in achieving a more effective half halt and a smoother halt. Remember that Joseph Pilates wanted the minimum of effort for the maximum effect.

### Experiment with downward transitions

At the walk, maintain the Basic Dressage Position (Open-Leg Rocker Position) with the least amount of muscle tension needed. To halt your horse, increase the effort of your stomach moving farther in and up while increasing the pulling back and down of your shoulders. Remember how you placed your back on the wall in the Wall Exercise in Chapter Five (Figure 5-9). As you do this, ever so slightly scoop your bottom as if to walk the hind legs forward under your seat and then stop the motion of the seat by pulling your stomach in again. See if you can stop your horse without using the reins. At first you may have to use your reins with the action of your Powerhouse. When the horse halts, be sure to release your stomach slightly but keep a light engagement of the bottom. If you release the stomach completely without the light engagement of the gluteals, you will probably fall forward. Experiment with just how much muscle engagement is needed to achieve the halt.

Gradually, you can teach your horse to respond to your Powerhouse muscles and save your rein aids for other cues. When you can use your Powerhouse to bring your horse from walk to halt, try the same experiment for performing a half halt or any type of downward transition. The muscle actions should be the same, however the difference will be in the amount of effort required.

Downward transitions from the canter will require the same directions as above. However the asymmetry of the body position during the canter will involve more attention to the isolation of the core/trunk muscles during the downward transition.

### EXPERIMENT WITH DOWNWARD TRANSITIONS FROM THE CANTER

While on the right lead canter, the right bottom (gluteus) and right shoulder (mid and lower trapezius) will be isolated and engaged more in order to keep the right seat bone forward and the right shoulder back. To bring a horse down from, for example, the right lead canter, the rider should sit the left seat bone down into the saddle. This is easily accomplished by releasing the extra muscular effort of the isolated right bottom. With this release you will find your seat bones drop evenly into the saddle. This drop into the saddle, combined with the above directions for downward transitions, should bring the horse to the trot or walk with less dependency on the reins.

### *THOUGHTS ON REIN-BACK*

When learning to back a horse, most riders are taught to lean forward to lighten the seat while pulling back on the reins. While this is effective, it is not the most efficient way to ask a horse to rein-back. Instead, lighten your seat by engaging your inner thighs and bottom muscles ever so slightly. The lift of your stomach up the spine will help lift your seat off the horse's back. While doing so, pull the stomach back farther than normal. Feel the energy of the whole back moving backward by pressing your shoulders farther back and down. You may find that, eventually, you can teach your horse to perform a rein-back by just pulling in your stomach. Then, to stop the horse from backing, release the muscle tension.

# POSTING TROT

In Training Level and most of First Level, as well as on young horses, riders post the trot. If one were to see the posting trot of a well-accomplished rider, it would look as though her shoulders and hands were staying in one place while her hips rise up and forward toward her hands and then gently move back down into the saddle. The rider has stabilized her Box. She can post by pivoting off her knees by extending her hip while leaving her lower leg long and loose. In contrast, a less experienced rider will try to post the trot by gripping with her lower legs for stability and pitching her whole body forward with her hips still in a flexed or decreased angle position. To create a more effective posting trot, try the following experiment:

### EXPERIMENT WITH POSTING TROT

For the posting trot, you will need to remember the "Single Leg Kick" exercise in Chapter 5 (Figure 5-6). Although this exercise was performed while lying on the stomach, the action of the bottom pushing the hip bones into the mat as the stomach pulled in and up is very much the same musculature needed for posting. Feel how the engagement of your bottom will send your hips forward toward your hands and the pommel of the saddle. Along with this action, feel your back against the wall as in the Wall Exercise (Figure 5-9). Maintain your shoulders and whole back on the wall by bringing your abdominals in and up. Keep the feeling of your shoulders moving down to meet your stomach in your lower back to help anchor your shoulder girdle down. Recall the feeling of your armpits moving down to your waistline from the Wall Arm Circles exercise to help you feel your bent elbows still at your side. Stilling your shoulders and elbows should enable you to keep your hands quiet as you post. With your Box held strongly in one place by the work of the Powerhouse and Box muscles, you should be able to achieve a more efficient posting trot.

# SITTING TROT

Sitting the trot is a major step in the dressage rider's training. Learning to sit the trot can be challenging, especially if the horse is not truly round and engaged. When an inexperienced rider tries to sit the trot, most often both horse and rider are jarred by the lack of harmony between the horse's back and the rider's seat. This jarring can create a juggling act for the horse. Now there is not just one mass on top of his back: there are many moving parts bouncing around creating worry and tension. This usually causes him to hollow his back even more.

The rider who cannot hold herself together in one strong but supple piece has no chance of trying to engage the horse in this situation. However, if the rider can hold herself in one solid but supple piece, the horse has less of a balancing act and, therefore, can relax and happily carry the rider on his rounded back.

## EXPERIMENT WITH SITTING TROT

To attain a strong but supple and dynamic position on a horse while sitting the trot, the rider has to recall the Basic Dressage Position (the Open Leg Rocker) and combine it with varying degrees of the Rolling Back (Figure 4-3). In the Rolling Back, the lower back is actively curling down toward the ground (collecting) and then releasing back slightly to a less curled position (engaged but lengthened). Combine this dynamic movement of the lower back with the lift of the upper body in the Open Leg Rocker. Feel your shoulders (mid and lower trapezius) engage, pulling back and down while your armpits move toward your waistline, stretching and stabilizing the rider's shoulders and elbows downward. Feel your upper thighs wrapping with judicious use of your bottom scooping and "rescooping" with each stride. By remaining stabilized in one place and in one piece, the horse will be encouraged to stay directly under you and begin to carry you with less tension. Experiment with how much or how little muscle tension is needed to accomplish this movement. Remember: too much muscle tension will create stiffness, which leads to jarring. Too little tension makes it impossible for the horse to carry the rider.

## *THOUGHTS ON LENGTHENING AND COLLECTION*

To help the lengthening and collection of horse in sitting trot, or in any gait, experiment with lengthening and collecting your own spine to ask the horse for these movements. Experimenting with this while mounted will require that you have mastered the full articulation of your spine. If you have performed the Rolling Back and the Roll Up from Chapter 4 and the Arching in Chapter 6 with success, you should be able to use these exercises in varying degrees to help your horse lengthen and collect his spine.

To ask your horse to lengthen, allow your own spine to lengthen and lift more. Using the Arching exercise (Figure 6-7), feel the lift in your sternum while maintaining the length in your spine by use of your Powerhouse. Your face will not turn upward toward the sky, but your focus will lift slightly as you look across the arena to the endpoint of the lengthening. Anchor this lift of your upper body with the increased use of your Powerhouse. Scoop your stomach in and up, squeeze your bottom and wrap your inner thighs to encourage your horse to move forward. Feel your seat bones pointing even more in the direction of your horse's head. This is the driving seat needed for lengthenings.

When you want your horse to collect, think of the directions for the downward transition first. Then continue to collect your spine by pulling your center of gravity closer to you by engaging your stomach further to stabilize and still your lower back. Keep your upper back engaged by using your shoulders back and down. Use your bottom and upper thighs as you did for the upward transitions, as needed, to keep the horse moving forward into collection.

# CIRCLING

To create and keep bend in a horse, you need to keep your shoulders and hips in line with the shoulders and hips of your horse. Since many dressage figures are based on circles, it is essential that the rider understand how to create a body position that aids and keeps the horse in a bend. The position must be strong, but not stiff, in order to maintain the flow of the horse's forward movement. Circles from 20 meters to voltes can be improved by thinking about exactly how your body needs to be stabilized during a circle.

### EXPERIMENT WITH CIRCLES

For this experiment, you will refer back to the Saw (Figure 5-3) and Twisting (Figure 6-6) exercises. Also refer to the Side Bend (Figure 5-14). The rider will be executing the first part of the Saw or the Twisting to ask the horse to execute the Side Bend.

Picture the bend of your horse's body and imagine his hips anchoring one end of the bend and the shoulders moving away from that to create the arch in his trunk just as you did when you performed the Side Bend. In order to help your horse anchor his hips, the rider must anchor her hips. To do this, use the Saw exercise where you must keep both seat bones firmly planted. The slight scoop in the pelvis from using the Powerhouse will help you do this. From there, lift your stomach in and up and rotate or twist your spine at your waist. You will feel your ribs turning above the pelvis, which is kept securely anchored in the saddle by the scoop of your bottom. By creating and maintaining this active posture, you are, in essence, keeping your shoulders and hips in line with your horse's body on a bend.

Tracking right, see if you can guide your horse onto a circle by merely twisting your spine to the right as described above. Be sure your shoulders are level, staying parallel to the hipbones. Use more or less twist to ask for smaller or larger circles. Keep your stomach engaged and your chest lifted as your spine turns. To return to a straight line, return your rib cage back to center. Reverse directions for a turn to the left. Experiment with how much twist is needed to create and maintain the size of the circle you want.

# SHOULDER-IN

As you move up the levels, movements get more complex. The shoulder-in requires the horse to travel on three tracks. The back legs are on two tracks, and the shoulder moves the front legs one track to the horse's inside, creating a third track for the inside foreleg. To bring the horse's shoulders in, you must ask the horse to take the first step toward a 10-meter circle. If you have already experimented with using the Saw or Twist to make a circle, try the following:

### EXPERIMENT WITH SHOULDER-IN
Using the Saw/Twist exercise as described in the above experiment, ask your horse to take one step toward the path of a circle while traveling right. This puts the horse in the shoulder-in position. The muscles needed to ask the horse for the first step onto the circle must now dynamically change in order to keep him traveling in shoulder-in as opposed to circling. To do this, you must maintain the twist in your body to the right, keep both seat bones anchored in the saddle and send the horse forward in the shoulder-in position by using your bottom.

To maintain the twisting of your trunk, you must continually pull your stomach in and up. Your chest will feel lifted, and your shoulders will remain parallel with the horse's shoulders. Engage your right mid and lower trapezius even more. Feel it continually moving back and down to meet your stomach in your lower back. While doing this you will notice that your hands will move to the inside as the muscular action of the shoulders will keep your elbows still at your waistline as your upper body twists from the waistline.

As your upper body twists to the right, just as in the Saw, you will notice that the natural tendency is for your left seat bone to come off the saddle. To counter this, keep your Powerhouse scoop with your bottom. Then, to send the horse forward down the side of the arena in shoulder-in, increase the use of the one-legged wrapping of the right leg that created the first step onto the circle. Your right gluteus and the back of your right upper thigh muscle wrapping around from back to front will actively engage and push your horse forward in the shoulder-in position. You will feel this as the action of a one-legged wringer washing machine (Figure 2-7).

This dynamic use of the Powerhouse muscles will enable you to keep your horse moving forward in shoulder-in. Experiment with just how much effort is needed to start and then maintain the horse moving in the shoulder-in down the track. To come out of the shoulder-in, release the extra muscle effort.

## THOUGHTS ON LEG YIELD

To help a horse travel in a straight path, it is essential that the rider be able to sit squarely on her horse. By practicing the Basic Dressage Position, the rider will not only be more able to do this on a horse that is standing still, but also be able to maintain this squareness in the saddle while the horse walks, trots and canters. To ask a horse to remain straight and move sideways at the same time is a challenge. Often the rider is tempted to lean either toward or away from the direction of the leg yield in order to make her horse move sideways. For example, if the rider is tracking right and wants to leg yield left, she may lean to the right in order to put force into her right leg to move the horse to the left. Or the rider may tilt to the left, trying to put more weight in the left stirrup so the horse is forced to move left to carry the weight of the rider.

To create a more harmonious leg yield, try holding your body more square by using your Powerhouse and Box muscles. To leg yield to the left, engage only the right bottom and use the wrapping of the right upper thigh to indicate to the horse to move both sideways and forward. Experiment with this to see if you can create a horse that is more responsive to your seat in order to execute a leg yield.

# HAUNCHES-IN AND HALF PASS

Just as in shoulder-in, haunches-in and half pass require that the rider maintain the horse on three tracks, and, just as in shoulder-in and circling, the rider needs to keep her shoulders and hips aligned with the shoulders and hips of her horse. However, the opposite of shoulder-in, the haunches-in and half pass require the horse to travel on three tracks with the front legs on two tracks and the haunches toward the inside creating a third track with the inside hind leg. The exercise that can help immensely with both of these movements is the Chest Expansion (Figure 5-16). More easily explained in half pass, you can use the same ideas to experiment with haunches-in on the track.

To perform a half pass, riders are often instructed to sit with the outside seat bone closer to the middle of the saddle and point the outside elbow in the direction they have come from. For the rider to do this, a dynamic stabilization of the Box is necessary. As the horse's hips move diagonally and forward, the rider's hips must also move diagonally and forward without allowing the shoulders to tilt or collapse. With the use of the bottom and the stabilization required of the Chest Expansion, these ideas for performing a half pass become much clearer.

## EXPERIMENT WITH HALF PASS

Think back to how your body felt while performing the Chest Expansion in Chapter 5 (See Figure 5-16). Chest Expansion requires you to pull your shoulders back and down as you pull your arms (hence elbows) behind you without allowing your ribs to splay forward. Your Powerhouse muscles must be totally engaged to do this while breathing in expands the chest. To use this exercise to help the half pass, you will be performing a one-sided Chest Expansion in conjunction with a one-sided, more engaged bottom.

When starting a half pass, it is essential that you keep your Box square by using your Powerhouse and trunk muscles. To ask for the half pass while tracking left, as you round the short side of the arena, expand only your right chest so that your right elbow comes back slightly behind you. This creates the idea of the elbow pointing in the direction from which you came. Do not allow your ribs to splay forward. When you pull your right shoulder back, you will probably find that your ribs will want to move to the left and forward and/or you may want to lean back and collapse to the right. Avoid this evasion by keeping your left shoulder back and down meeting your stomach in your lower back to stabilize the torso. Also, be sure your right hip does not pull backward. Rather, engage the right gluteus more as you scoop and drive the horse diagonally forward. This will create the outside seat bone moving closer to the middle of the saddle. You will need to keep your stomach engaged as if you had a corset on to counteract the evasions of the one-sided Chest Expansion.

Experiment with just how much muscle effort is required to begin and maintain the half pass. Release the Chest Expansion and extra use of the one gluteal action to travel straight again. Reverse above direction of the one-sided Chest Expansion to experiment with the half pass while tracking right.

## HAUNCHES-IN

Usually the movement learned before the half pass is the haunches-in. This is the same three-track movement as described for the half-pass. The half pass is basically haunches-in ridden on the diagonal. Experiment with the same directions for half pass. You will not have the easier cue of pointing the elbow in the direction from which you came. To help establish a haunches-in on the long side of the arena, experiment with the following.

## Experiment with Haunches-In

While tracking left, as you come out of the corner on the short side anchor your shoulders down to meet your stomach in your lower back. Use your Powerhouse and feel that you are wearing a corset to hold your ribs in place while you perform the one-sided Chest Expansion. You will feel the action of the Chest Expansion with your right elbow moving slightly behind your shoulder and scoop the right bottom more. Experiment with how much or how little effort you need or can use to create the haunches-in. Release the one-sided musculature and return to the Basic Dressage Position to continue straight along the track.

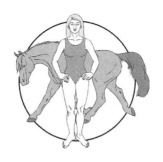

# APPENDICES

## UNDERSTANDING STYLISTIC APPROACHES TO PILATES TRAINING

With most disciplines, there are various stylistic approaches to training that stem from an original teaching. Yoga, ballet, dressage and other disciplines have developed over many years and, in each one, a student can find dozens of instructors who all purport to teach the discipline. The Pilates Method has not been immune from this spawning of approaches that are gleaned from the original idea.

When researching or doing a Web search for Pilates, a person find; a lizzying array of approaches to the exercise method created by Joseph Pilates. While some of the approaches may be based on the true work of Pilates, many programs have been created by people who do not have the in-depth training or knowledge to truly pass on the work of Joseph Pilates. These, perhaps, well-intentioned persons, will attempt to teach Pilates, but the Pilates taught will undoubtedly have little resemblance to the real Pilates work.

The original teachings of Joseph Pilates were entrusted to Romana Kryzanowska when Joseph Pilates died in the late 1960s. Pilates left Ms. Kryzanowska his archives, which included writings, photographs and films in which he documented his work over the years. Also, Romana's years of working at Joseph Pilates' side ensures that her knowledge of the Pilates Method is as close to the original teachings as possible.

# HOW TO FIND A QUALIFIED, CERTIFIED INSTRUCTOR

The popularity of The Pilates Method, along with the different stylistic approaches to teaching Pilates, has brought numerous certification programs. These programs range from two-day certification courses to programs requiring 600—800 hours of training and apprenticeships. As in dressage, finding a competent instructor can be difficult. However just as the U.S. Dressage Federation has developed a rigorous instructor certification program to help people seeking solid dressage training find a qualified instructor, Romana Kryzanowska, the heir to the Pilates Method, has worked to preserve the original teachings of Joseph Pilates by creating a similar teacher certification course to help persons seeking to learn the work of Joseph Pilates to find qualified instruction.

Romana's Pilates, Inc. of New York, offers one of the most intensive teacher training programs in the world. The Romana's Pilates Independent Teacher Training courses are taught by Kryzanowska's appointed and Certified Level Three Instructors (certified to teach the equivalent of Training to Second Level), Level Two Instructors (certified to teach the equivalent of Training to Prix St. Georges) and the Level One master teachers, (certified to teach the equivalent of Training to Grand Prix). At the time this book was written, the Level One Master Teacher certification is limited to Kryzanowska and her daughter, Sari Mejia Santo.

The rigorous Romana's Pilates Independent Teacher Training program requires potential teachers to pass an assessment test performing at the intermediate level (or the equivalent of riding Second or Third Levels) in order to begin the program. Upon passing the assessment, the apprentice must take three intensive four- to five- day training courses while continuing to take their own private lessons with appropriate instructors. These training courses, Beginning, Intermediate, and Advanced Pilates Systems, are held over a period of six months, during which time the apprentice serves an apprenticeship with Level One, Level Two and Level Three instructors. This apprenticeship usually continues over a period of one year (approximately 800 hours) and includes observation hours, assisting teaching and apprentice teaching under supervision. The apprentice must test out of each course with both a written and practical exam. The final test, which leads to certification, is taken with either Kryzanowska or Santo, thus ensuring that the Master Teachers approve each certification candidate.

Because of this intensive training, instructors certified by Romana's Pilates are the most qualified to teach the Pilates Method. It is the author's recommendation that persons seeking to learn Pilates be advised to inform themselves as to their prospective instructor's qualifications to teach Pilates. For more information on Romana's Pilates certified instructors, visit the web site *www.romanaspilates.com.*

# ABOUT THE AUTHOR

Janice Dulak—dancer, teacher, choreographer and Level 2 Pilates instructor—has trained in Pilates with Romana Kryzanowska (heir to the Pilates Method) since 1989 when a knee injury threatened to end her performing career as a professional modern dancer. With improved body conditioning gained by Pilates, Ms. Dulak was able to continue dancing and teaching internationally. In 1993 Ms. Dulak was certified by Kryzanowska as a Pilates instructor and opened her first studio that year in Columbia, Missouri. During this time, Ms. Dulak served as chair of the dance department at Stephens College in Columbia for 10 years where she trained dancers in modern dance, choreography, improvisation and ballet as well as in the Pilates Method.

At the request of Romana Kryzanowska, Dulak undertook further training and received her Level Two instructor certification in 2000. This certification by Romana's Pilates Inc. of New York is held by only a handful of Pilates instructors. This certification qualifies Dulak to train Pilates instructors at seminars held at her studio (now The Pilates Center in Champaign, Illinois: *www.pilatesctr.com*) as well as at any national or international Romana's Pilates Training affiliate centers.

Janice Dulak has been riding dressage since 1995 and won a Gold Medal at First Level at the 2000 Show Me State Games in Columbia, Missouri. She rides her mare India at Second and Third Level and is currently starting her now 4-year old Oldenburg gelding, Rubaiyat, for a career in dressage at her and her husband's Amber Waves Farm in Champaign, Illinois. She trains in dressage with Terri Elsesser Stark and clinics regularly with David Blake, both USDF Gold medalists.

# ABOUT THE PHYSICAL THERAPIST

Katrin Haselbacher was born and raised in Zurich, Switzerland. She received her physical therapy degree at The University Hospital Zurich in 1999 and worked there for almost two years before coming to the United States in 2001. Since arriving in the United States, Ms. Haselbacher has worked as a physical therapist in both Champaign and Chicago, Illinois. She is currently working at the Rehabilitation Institute of Chicago.

# ABOUT THE ILLUSTRATOR

Eva Sandor became an illustrator at age 5, with the publication of dozens of her animal drawings in the form of a coloring book to benefit environmental causes. Throughout childhood, Ms. Sandor was fascinated with both animals and art, and continued to provide illustrations for many more publications; she took up art as a career and received her BFA from Carnegie-Mellon University in 1991 and her MFA from The University of Wisconsin-Madison in 1997. While in graduate school, Ms Sandor discovered dressage and was immediately hooked. She and her husband own one horse and lease another, and despite living in a big city (Chicago) they manage to commute to the barn where they ride almost every evening.

# ABOUT THE PHOTOGRAPHER

Andy Ducette is an artist from Minnesota and is currently pursuing a graduate degree at the University of Illinois, Urbana-Champaign.

# ENDNOTES

1 Joeseph Pilates, "*Return to Life*," (U.S.A., 1960), 5.

2 George Russell, "*Keep Fit? Ape the Animals, Says the Gym Master*",  Sunday News, (26 May, 1963), 83

3 Marian Horosko, "*Pilates Power—All Over Warm-up Exercises: Part Four*," Dance Magazine, (February 1987), 82.

4 Hodges P.W. and Richardson C.A.,  "*Feedforward contraction of transversus abdominis is not influenced by the direction of arm movement*" Experimental Brain Research, (1997) 114: 362-370

# INDEX